A D V A

DRAG
TOUCH

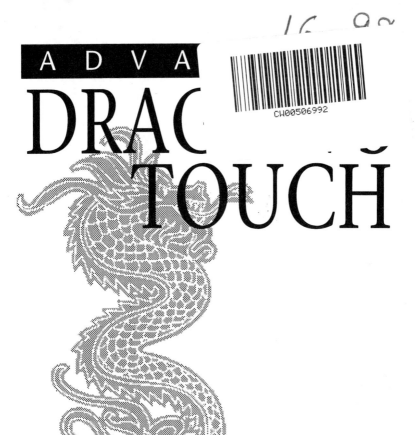

Master Hei Long

DRAGON'S TOUCH

20 Anatomical Targets and Techniques for Taking Them Out

PALADIN PRESS • BOULDER, COLORADO

Also by Master Hei Long:

Da Qiang Ji: Power Striking

Da Zhimingde: Striking Deadly Blows to Vital Organs

Danger Zones: Defending Yourself against Surprise Attack

Dragons Touch: Weaknesses of the Human Anatomy

Gouzao Gongji: Seven Neurological Attacks for Inflicting Serious Damage

Guge Gongji: Seven Primary Targets to Take Anyone Out of a Fight

Iron Hand of the Dragon's Touch: Secrets of Breaking Power

Master's Death Touch: Unarmed Killing Techniques

Master's Guide to Basic Self-Defense: Progressive Retraining of the Reflexive Response

21 Techniques of Silent Killing

Advanced Dragon's Touch:
20 Anatomical Targets and Techniques for Taking Them Out
by Master Hei Long

Copyright © 1995 by Master Hei Long

ISBN 0-87364-852-8

Printed in the United States of America

Published by Paladin Press, a division of
Paladin Enterprises, Inc., P.O. Box 1307,
Boulder, Colorado 80306, USA.
(303) 443-7250

Direct inquiries and/or orders to the above address.

Contents

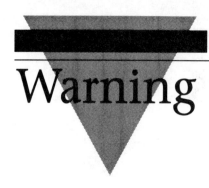

Warning

Some of the techniques depicted in this book are extremely dangerous. It is not the intent of the author, publisher, or distributors of this book to encourage readers to attempt any of these techniques without proper professional supervision and training. Attempting to do so can result in serious injury or death. Do not attempt any of these techniques without the supervision of a certified instructor.

The author, publisher, and distributors of this book disclaim any liability from any damages or injuries of any type that a reader or user of information contained herein may encounter from the use or misuse of said information. *This book is presented for academic study only.*

Introduction

The original *Dragons Touch* filled a vacuum in U.S. martial arts studies by focusing primarily on the anatomy and physiology of striking areas most commonly referred to as "pressure points." In that book, we studied 43 major pressure points of the body with a minimum analysis of the application of technique. Since then, *Guge Gongji, Gouzao Gongji,* and *Da Zhimingde* have been published, which focused on striking areas selected to fit into specific categories in terms of the physiological responses that would result from hitting them. Each of these studies met a need as well. *Advanced Dragon's Touch* will once again meet a demand—one fathered by an increasingly violent social order.

When the original *Dragons Touch* was published, carjacking was almost nonexistent, and assaults at ATMs were rare as well. As the variety of crimes expands, legislation to prohibit citizens from arming themselves is expanding also. Faced with this dilemma, people are turning toward alternative methods of defending themselves, their families, and their property. There are electronic weapons available, including shocking devices and alarms, but a defense that relies on a device of any kind is rendered useless if the victim doesn't have the time or opportunity to use it or if it fails to operate or is dropped in the scuffle. Reliance on one's own abilities is the most dependable self-defense device one can have.

Twenty anatomical targets have been selected and reviewed for this study, and the majority of the text is devoted to practical application. There are more than 50 techniques taught in this text, with the selected pressure points as targets of the counterstrikes. In addition, it includes a brief study of hand-weapon postures, focusing on some that may be familiar and some that may not. Study these closely: a weak striking instrument yields weak results.

CHAPTER ONE

Anatomical Weapons

The study of anatomical targets is complemented by a study of additional anatomical weapons. Small targets, especially those that are recessed, are most readily and effectively attacked with anatomical weapons whose points of contact are also relatively small or whose postures form a protuberance with which to strike.

The postures of anatomical weapons are significant in two ways. First is effectiveness. An improperly formulated weapon can result in "give" along any number of corresponding joints, cushioning the potential impact of the blow. Second, and perhaps of even greater importance, is that improperly formed weapons can be injured upon impact with the target. Open-hand weapons are most susceptible to these problems, though even closed-hand weapons can be injured when improperly applied. The wrists and thumb joints are usually the points of injury on closed-hand weapons. A study of the book *Iron Hand of the Dragon's Touch* will help prevent injury to anatomical weapons.

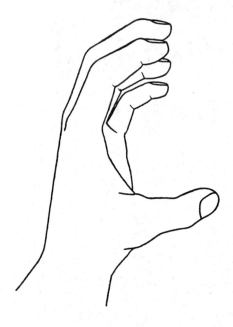

FIGURE 1

THE CLAW

The claw weapon's two uses are poking and grappling; its primary targets are the eyes, anterior neck region, and groin. Observe Figure 1. Open the hand and spread the fingers as wide as they will go comfortably. Hold the fingers, thumb, and wrist rigid throughout. The points of contact are the tips of the fingers and, in some applications, the fingers themselves.

In the second application, the claw is applied with a thrust into the face, the eyes being the intended target. In the second application, the center of the palm is used as a striking surface for soft targets, and the fingers are immediately clamped shut in a grappling motion. The anterior neck region is a prime target for this strike-and-grab application when used with a sweep or other type of takedown. Another target, the groin, is seen most

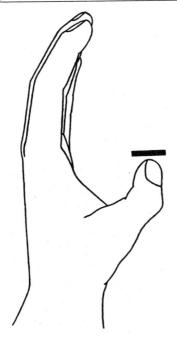

FIGURE 2

often as an initial loosening strike for defenses against such holds as bearhugs, headlocks, etc. It also works well with hand combinations, especially those that incorporate ducking or kneeling under incoming blows. The well-developed claw has a number of additional uses, including extracting bones from the body and tearing muscles from bones.

THE HOOK

The hook is also used as a poking instrument and has two primary targets—the eyes and anterior neck region. This weapon is not designed for grappling but solely for jabbing at small, soft targets. As in Figure 2, the fingers are held against each other, rigid and slightly bent, and the thumb is held slightly bent and away from the palm. The contact point is the tip of the

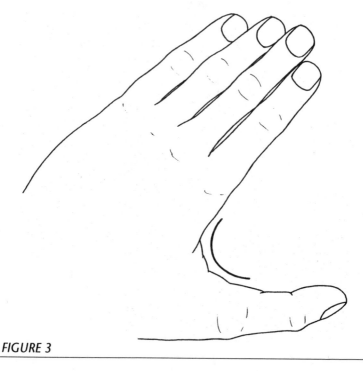

FIGURE 3

thumb. The hook is applied to both the eyes and anterior neck region with a thrusting motion. At close quar-
ters, the hook may be pushed into the eyes to break
holds and other types of traps.

TIGER MOUTH

The tiger mouth has one target: the anterior neck
region. Its very design facilitates its application to the
target even for opponents with very short necks (see fig.
3). Lay your forearm and hand palm-down on a flat surface. Hold the fingers straight and together, and spread
the thumb to its limit from the hand. When you have
done this, rotate the hand to the outside of the forearm
until the wrist locks. Hold all corresponding muscles
rigid from the elbow through the fingers. The contact
point is indicated by the half-moon line between the

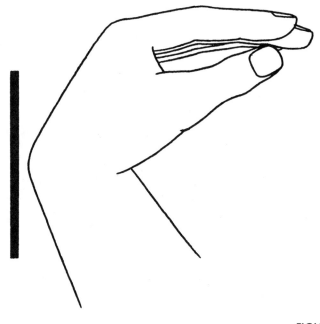

FIGURE 4

thumb and index fingers. Like the hook and claw forma-
tions, the tiger mouth is applied to its target in a thrusting fashion but may also be applied with a bent-arm
sweeping motion.

CHICKEN WRIST

The chicken wrist is a great deal more dense than
one might imagine and forms a very hard, solid striking surface. The targets for this weapon are numerous.
Of the 20 pressure points we will be attacking in this
study, 12 are structurally susceptible to the snapping
impact of the chicken wrist. They are the fossa temporalis, septal cartilage, cervical vertebrae, temporomandibular joint, tip of the mandible, carotid plexus,
anterior neck region, sternum, heart, solar plexus, ribs,
and groin. As shown in Figure 4, bend the wrist inward

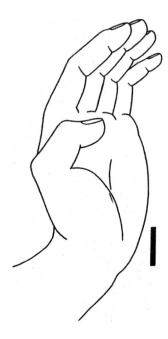

FIGURE 5

as far as it will go, hold the fingers and the thumb straight, together, and rigid. The striking surface is the outer point of the wrist. The chicken wrist is a hard weapon and can therefore be applied to both hard and soft targets. The chicken wrist approaches its target with a trajectory almost identical to that of a backhand but with a degree of straight-line push.

The weapon is best suited as a lead-in strike off a crossing palm block and is deceptively applied from the waist on a rising plane to such targets as the tip of the mandible and the anterior neck region.

THE PALM

The palm strike is a versatile weapon that may be applied vertically both upward and downward, horizontally with a snap or a sweep, and also with a straight-line

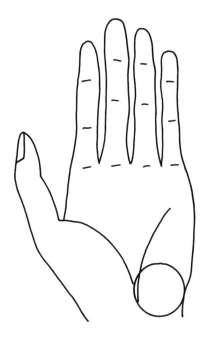

FIGURE 6

thrust. Of the 22 targets selected for this study, only the eyes, anterior neck region, and coccyx are not recommended for this blow.

As shown in Figure 5, pull the hand back as far as it will go and hold the fingers only as straight as necessary to keep them from folding inward. There are two correct thumb positions for the palm strike. One is depicted in Figure 5, the other in Figure 6. Choosing which to use is a matter of personal preference. You will want to be aware of an opponent wearing loose clothing: if the thumb became entangled it could be sprained or broken rather easily. The points of contact for this weapon are denoted by the circle in Figure 6 and the bar in Figure 5. The palm strike is probably the most damage-resistant of all the upper-body weapons and develops for breaking sooner than the others with a minimum of risk of injury.

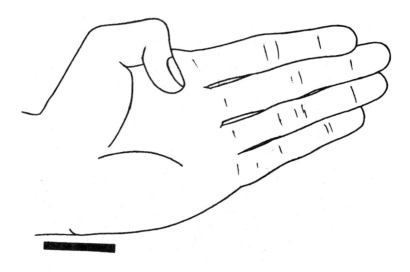

FIGURE 7

THE SUTO

The suto is both a speed and power weapon. It is easily applied with controlled depth or full penetration, horizontally in a palm-up or palm-down position, or with a downward vertical stroke. Its prime targets are the fossa temporalis, carotid plexus, anterior neck region, base of the cranium, and brachial plexus. Observe Figures 7 and 8. The suto is formed by either spreading the fingers and bending them slightly, or by holding the fingers straight and slightly overlapping them. The thumb is folded and pulled down while being kept on the thumb side of the hand. Place the hand and arm on a flat surface and rotate the hand toward the thumb as far as it will go. This is the proper posture for the suto. The point of contact is denoted in both illustrations.

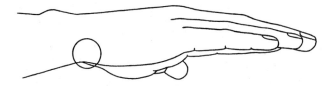

FIGURE 8

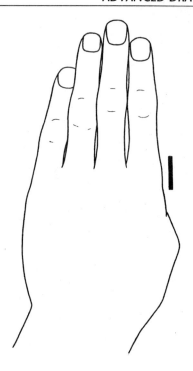

FIGURE 9

INSIDE SUTO

The inside suto is designed as a weapon of power. It uses a long-stroke approach and relies on centrifugal force to generate its impact power. It is not generally applied with controlled penetration, as in a snap, but rather is driven into the target, allowing the target itself to stop its progression.

Note that in the suto shown in Figure 9, the thumb is pulled inward and away from the striking surface. This requires the thumb to cross the palm and be held firmly in that position. In Figure 10, the striking surface is circled. Because the arm is extended in the strike, the inside suto works well to strike an opponent from his outside, and since it is at its peak of power while the arm is extended, the inside suto makes an excellent weapon in combination with outside blocks and slips. Keep in

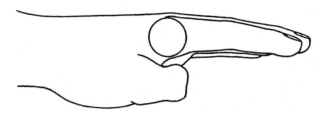

FIGURE 10

mind that though the arm is fully extended, the elbow is not locked in the open position. Keep a slight bend in the elbow to prevent hyperextending it.

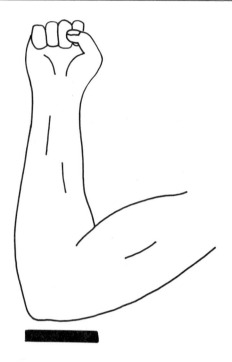

FIGURE 11

ELBOW STRIKES

Elbow strikes are comparatively short-stroke blows that are best suited for close-contact fighting, though they may be initiated from a longer range by using a gap-closing step to bring a selected target within the required proximity. Elbows are best suited for larger, solid targets that can absorb the power of the drive, such as the ribs, heart, sternum, and cervical and thoracic vertebrae, but smaller, softer areas may be targeted as well.

Figure 11 shows the bottom elbow-striking area; Figure 12 shows the forward striking area. The position in Figure 11 would be applied in a downward vertical stroke to such targets as the suprasternal notch or, when an opponent is bent over, to the vertebrae. This striking area may also be used horizontally to the east, west, and south gates. The position in Figure 12 may be applied in

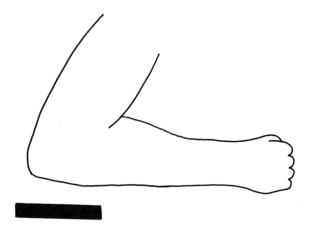

FIGURE 12

an upward vertical stroke to the tip of the mandible or in a forward horizontal stroke to a number of other target areas.

The biggest advantage of elbow strikes can be realized in a close-quarter situation. Elbow power is at a premium when you are chest to chest with an opponent, while the longer-stroke weapons such as sutos, backhands, and straight-line punches are crowded and comparatively ineffective.

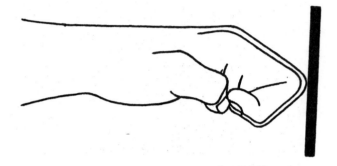

FIGURE 13

THE FOREFIST

The very appearance of this weapon—and its position in relation to the target in Figure 13—makes it evident that it was designed to fit into small areas, approaching its target with a straight-line thrust or a thrusting jab. Its narrow posture makes it especially effective against the anterior neck region, where an approaching weapon would have to fit under the chin.

The forefist is basically a half-closed fist. The thumb is folded and pulled toward the palm until the nails of the thumb and index finger are touching. The point of contact is the second knuckle of the middle finger. The fingers, thumb, and wrist are held rigid throughout when delivering the blow.

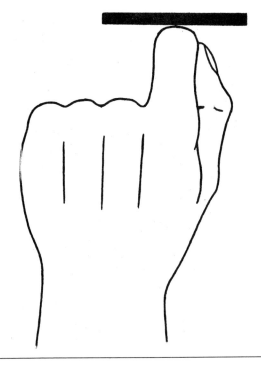

FIGURE 14

ONE-KNUCKLE FIST

The one-knuckle fist is a very firm, solid poking weapon designed primarily to be used on small targets. Its meager striking surface, coupled with its straight-line, thrusting power source, makes it a potentially lethal weapon when applied to the properly selected targets. The temples, carotid plexus, anterior neck region, suprasternal notch, and eyes are the primary targets. The sternum, solar plexus, and ribs are secondary targets.

Make a fist and then extend the index finger to the half point, as shown in Figure 14. Press the thumb against the partially extended finger to support it. When using this weapon, hold the hand rigid through the wrist. The one-knuckle fist has the advantage of being effective at both long and short range from a variety of chamber positions.

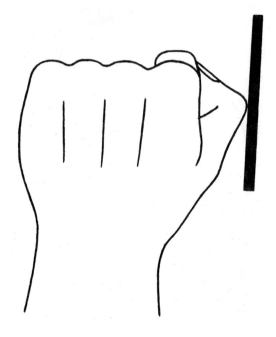

FIGURE 15

THE THUMB FIST

As is the one-knuckle fist, the thumb fist is a solid poking weapon with a small striking surface. This weapon, however, is designed to utilize the centrifugal power principle and, consequently, will have much greater power. Again, your primary targets will be the temples, carotid plexus, anterior neck region, and eyes. The sternum, solar plexus, and ribs will be secondary targets.

Form a fully closed fist and then bring the thumb to its side, pressing the tip of the thumb against the second joint of the index finger, as shown in Figure 15. The second knuckle of the thumb is the striking surface. The two advantages to using this weapon are its focused striking surface and centrifugal power source. Being struck in the ribs or sternum with this weapon is similar

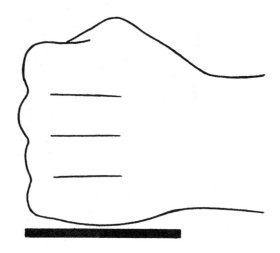

FIGURE 16

to being jabbed with the end of a pool stick or comparable instrument.

THE HAMMER FIST

The hammer fist, or "hand hammer," is a multipurpose striking weapon that works well on both hard and soft targets, and it may be used with a number of power sources, including centrifugal force. The hammer fist quickly responds to conditioning and is a popular selection for breaking practice.

Close the hand to a full fist, holding the muscles of the hand, wrist, and forearm tightly (fig. 16). The striking area is basically the same as with the suto, but the entire bottom of the fist may be used and responds well to conditioning. The septal cartilage, suprasternal notch, sternum, and heart are typical targets for the

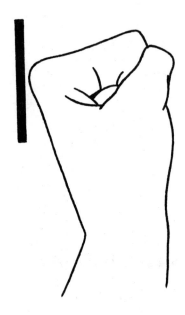

FIGURE 17

hand hammer when confronting an upright opponent.
The cervical and thoracic vertebrae, brachial plexus, and
biceps are also good targets for the various applications
of this weapon.

THE BACKHAND

The backhand is among the most useful of the
upper body weapons. It has multiple power sources
that range from the speed snap to the full 360-degree
centrifugal force application, it has two completely different contact areas and corresponding designs, and it
is as well suited to a diversionary lead strike as to a one-
stroke knockdown or finishing blow. Observe Figures
17 and 18. Figure 17 shows the two-knuckle application. The hand is tightly closed into a fist with the
wrist bent back slightly. The contact area is the first

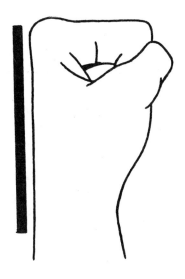

FIGURE 18

two knuckles. This application is designed for focused contact to cut or break large targets or to strike such small, recessed targets such as the eyes and fossa temporalis. In Figure 18, the entire flat of the back of the hand is used. This design is best suited for targets that are damaged by deep penetration, such as the carotid plexus, anterior neck region, and cervical vertebrae. The ribs, heart, solar plexus, and groin are also suitable targets for this weapon.

THE FULL FIST

The fully closed fist, in a straight-line or other application, is generally the first weapon taught in most martial arts systems but is omitted in advanced training. Its dense posture makes it suitable for literally any anatomical target it can fit into, and its variable approach trajec-

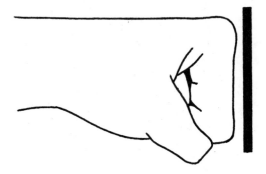

FIGURE 19

tories render it useful in most combative situations. The full-turn punch depicted in Figure 19 is designed to make contact with the first two knuckles of the fist. As with the backhand, the concentrated contact points focus the sum of the force into a smaller area, resulting in a cutting and breaking effect. The half-turn punch depicted in Figure 20 uses the entire face of the fist to cover larger areas and to apply the controlled penetration concussion effect, which works well on subcutaneous targets such as the heart, solar plexus, and kidneys.

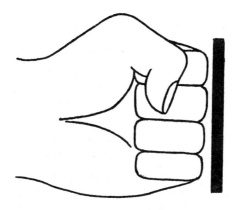

FIGURE 20

CHAPTER TWO

Pressure Points #1 through #6

In this chapter we will study the first six pressure points and applied techniques for directing attacks to these areas. These facial targets are the temple, eyes, ears, septal cartilage, mandible, and tip of the mandible. Two of them are potentially lethal, and though it is not suggested that non-lethal targets be studied with less seriousness, obviously it is more important to have a thorough understanding of life-threatening target areas so you can both use them effectively when necessary and avoid them when prudent.

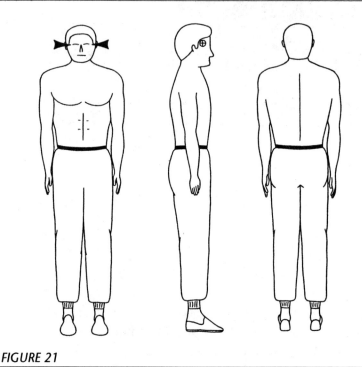

FIGURE 21

PRESSURE POINT #1: THE TEMPLE

Observe Figure 21, and reach up to the side of your head next to your eyes. If you place your fingers into the depression of the temple and press gently, you will detect a pulse and a basically soft area surrounded by bone.

Now observe Figures 22 through 25. In Figure 22, the meningeal artery is shown at the point where it surfaces in the tempa fossil. Look at the cross section of the skull in Figure 23. Locate the sphenoid and the area denoted as the temple. Figure 24 is a more specific illustration of the sphenoid. Pay special attention to the areas designated as the great wings and the small wings. It is the tips of the great wings that extend near the surface of the side of the skull, as noted by the blackened area in Figure 25.

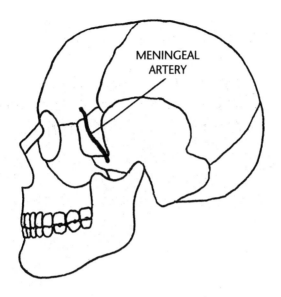

MENINGEAL
ARTERY

FIGURE 22

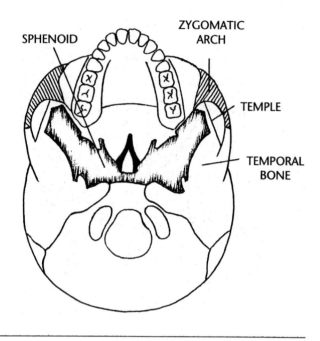

FIGURE 23

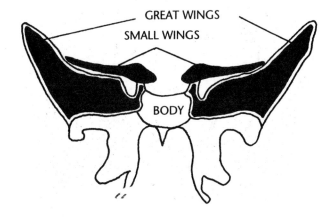

GREAT WINGS

SMALL WINGS

BODY

FIGURE 24

Go back to Figure 23 and note the space between the tips of the great wings of the sphenoid and the adjoining areas denoted as the temple. The tempa fossil (surrounding bony formation) is formed at the bottom by the junction of the temporal bone and the zygomatic arch, and the frontal, parietal, and adjacent portions of the temporal bone form the top and sides. It is the space between the tips of the great wings of the sphenoid and the surface of the temple that allows the meningeal artery to pass outside the protection of the skull within the tempa fossil.

Striking this area with a high-impact blow could be lethal if the weapon's striking surface is small and its impact is not dispersed by the tempa fossil. An uninhibited, high-powered blow could break the tips of the great wings, forcing them into the brain and causing instantaneous death. A blow of lesser force could still be lethal if

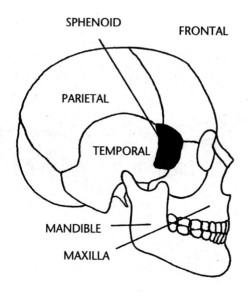

FIGURE 25

it was powerful enough to rupture the meningeal artery. The incoming blow would trap the artery between the striking surface and the tips of the great wings, creating a squeeze-crush effect. The rupturing of the meningeal artery would cause compression of the brain.

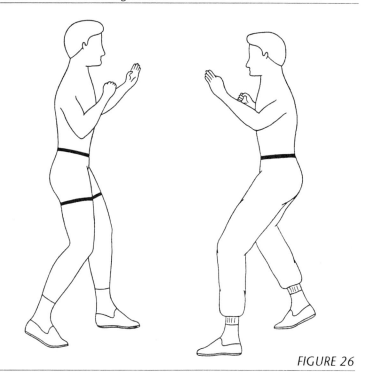

FIGURE 26

Practical Application Technique #1

Observe Figures 26 through 29. In Figure 26, both you (in long pants) and your opponent are in standard ready positions. In Figure 27, your opponent begins an advancing roundhouse punch, and you shuffle-step forward and stop the blow with an inside suto block. As shown in Figure 28, immediately upon the block-strike contact, you extend the blocking arm over the punching arm and force your arm downward in a circular motion. Form a thumb fist with the left hand, and with an upward, circular drive, strike the temple while rotating your entire body in the direction of the blow (fig. 29). This is your optimum-power centrifugal force drive, which was discussed in detail in *Da Qiang Ji: Power Striking.*

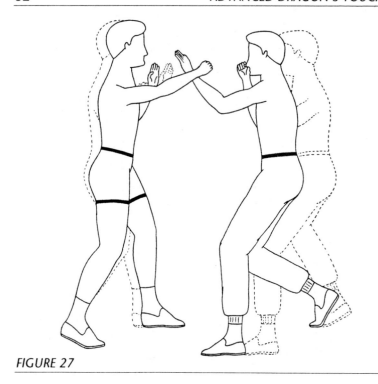

FIGURE 27

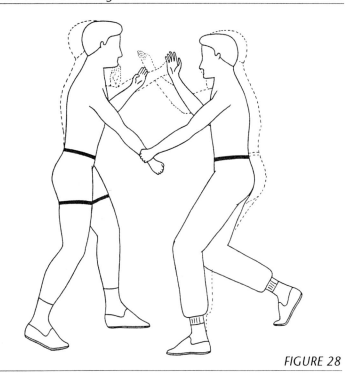

FIGURE 28

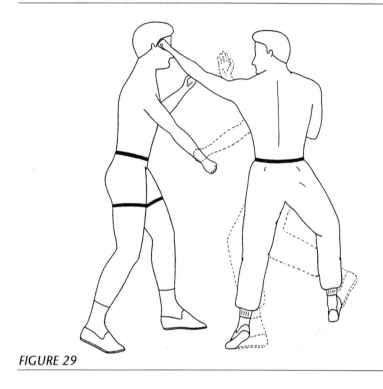

FIGURE 29

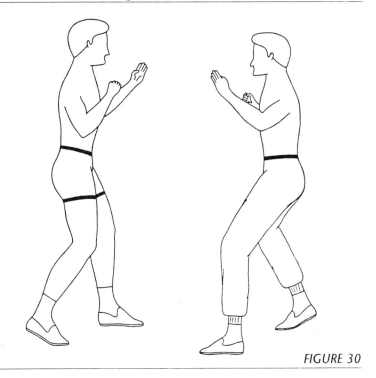

FIGURE 30

Practical Application Technique #2

You begin in a ready stance (fig. 30), and your opponent advances with a face-high vertical jab, which you
will block with an inside suto block (fig. 31). Observe
Figures 32 and 33. When you block the lead punch, the
opponent immediately follows with a low gate punch.
Your second block, using the same hand that blocked
the first blow, arcs downward, catching the incoming
punch at the wrist. You chamber a wide horizontal palm
blow simultaneously. Then, using a drive from the
upper body and a rotation of your stance, you drive the
horizontal palm strike into your opponent's temple, as
in Figure 34.

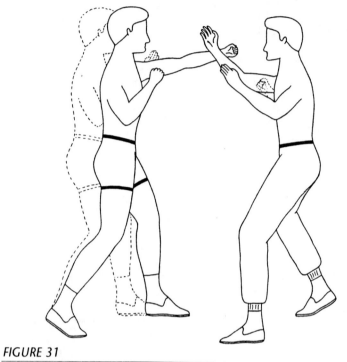

FIGURE 31

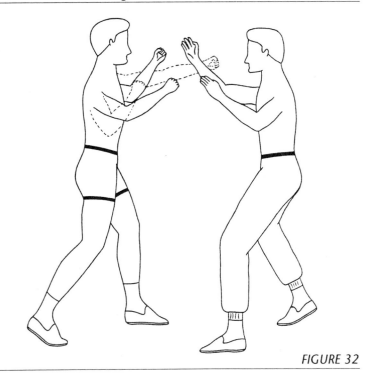

FIGURE 32

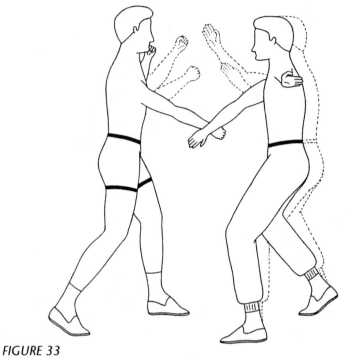

FIGURE 33

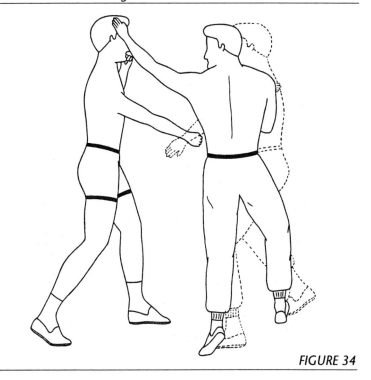

FIGURE 34

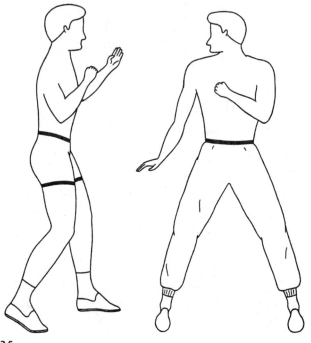

FIGURE 35

Practical Application Technique #3

In this technique you are intentionally leaving your
hands positioned low on your body to draw a blow to
the face (fig. 35). The stance is solid and intended to
reinforce quick upper body movement. In Figure 36, as
your opponent lunges in with a left straight-line punch
to your face, you lean your upper-body back from the
incoming blow and chamber your right backhand. In
Figure 37, you snap your upper body back to its original
position while thrusting your backhand into your opponent's temple on the way. Use your returning upper-
body movement to enhance the power of the extending
backhand.

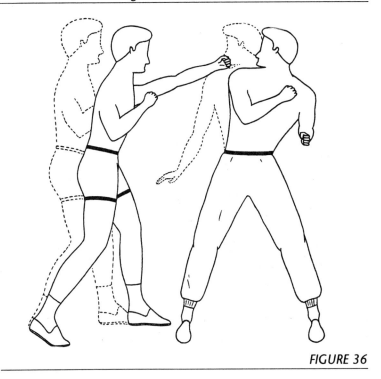

FIGURE 36

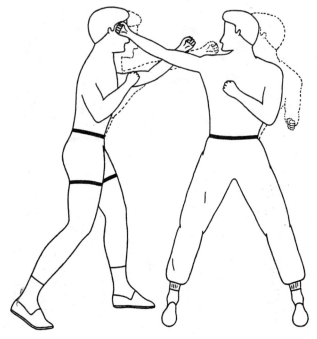

FIGURE 37

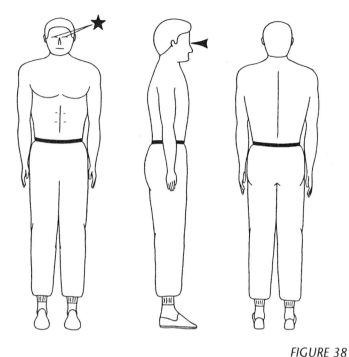

FIGURE 38

PRESSURE POINT #2: EYES

Observe Figure 38. The eyes are located on each side of the bridge of the nose, directly beneath the protection of the forehead. At one time or another, most people have had something as small as a grain of sand or a speck of dust in their eyes and have experienced the consequent discomfort, tearing, and pain associated with even minor contact to the eye. By examining the eyeball, one may better understand the dangers involved with contact to the eyes.

ORBITAL FISSURES

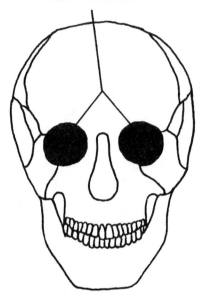

FIGURE 39

In Figure 39, the blackened areas in the skull depict those areas where the bony portion of the face ends, leaving the orbital fissures in which the eyeballs rest.

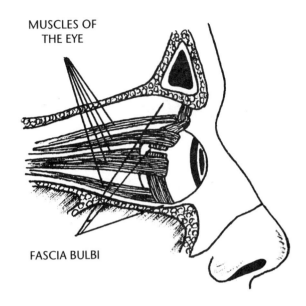

MUSCLES OF
THE EYE

FASCIA BULBI

FIGURE 40

The cut-away view of the face in Figure 40 shows how most of the eyeball sits back in the orbital fissure. The fascia bulbi, a thin membrane within the fatty lining of the orbit, holds the eyeball in place along with the muscles of the eye. The muscles that help hold the eyeball in place also control its movement and have elastic properties that allow the eyeball to be displaced outside the confines of the orbital fissure without being severed. The cross section depicted in Figure 41 illustrates the form and structure of the eyeball. The cornea is the outermost covering of the eye. Directly beneath the cornea is the anterior chamber, the pupil, surrounded by the iris and the lens. The posterior chambers of the eyeball are filled with a vitreous fluid that holds the eyeball in its spherical shape. If these chambers were penetrated, causing the fluid to leak out, the eyeball would collapse.

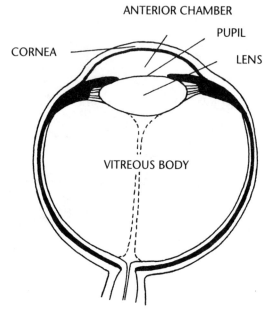

FIGURE 41

The most immediate dangers associated with strikes to the eyes are, of course, the partial or total loss of vision, whether temporary or permanent. The sensitivity of the eye, even to a touch or a light poke, makes it a preferred target.

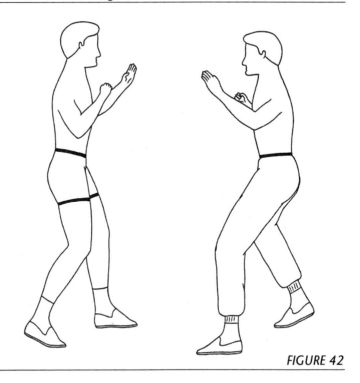

FIGURE 42

Practical Application Technique #4

In Figure 42, both you and your opponent are positioned in a ready stance. You will want to keep in mind that attacks to the eyes should invest speed over power. Since only a minimum amount of force and penetration is needed to injure the eyes, getting the blow to the target is your second priority; accuracy is, of course, the first. In Figure 43, your opponent is en route with a high right-handed punch to the face. Because you will be using a simultaneous block-and-strike technique, your movement will have no prestrike blocks or steps. In one quick, smooth motion (fig. 44), step to the outside of the incoming punch, guide it to the outside of your face, and snap a claw hand into your opponent's eyes.

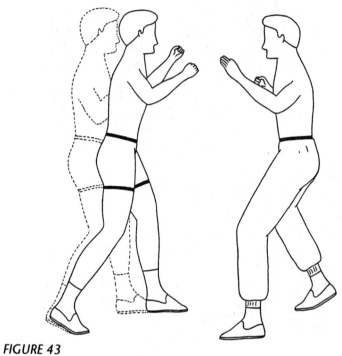

FIGURE 43

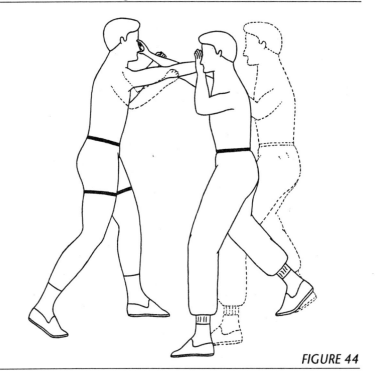

FIGURE 44

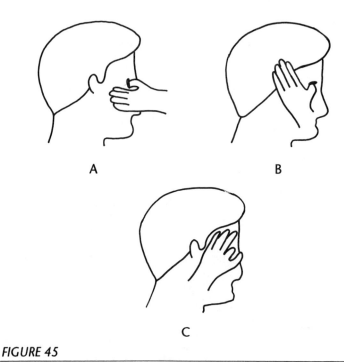

A   B

C

FIGURE 45

Practical Application Technique #5

The eyes are most useful as targets in clinch situations
when you can poke and scrape them. Many fights wind up
in grapples while the contenders are pushing, pulling,
falling to the ground, and reaching arm's length from their
bodies to generate enough power to land a hard punch.
Most often the opponent's head is within hand's reach,
and in fact it is very common for combatants to hold each
other around the neck, attempting to choke each other.
With half the strength it would take to effectively choke an
opponent, and with much quicker results, you can poke an
eye with a finger or simply scrape a finger across an eye,
causing considerable damage to your opponent. In Figure
45, A and B show the hand position to press forcefully or
poke an eye with a thumb, while C shows an index finger
application. These attacks are extremely effective during
most grappling situations.

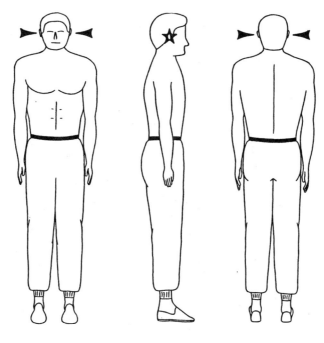

FIGURE 46

PRESSURE POINT #3: EARS

Observe Figure 46. As with the eyes, the ears need little analysis regarding location. Everyone knows where the ears are. However, most people do not realize their strategic value as a target. We will begin with an analysis of the ear's physical structure. Observe Figures 47 and 48. The external acoustic meatus is the canal leading into the ear. The tympanic membrane, more commonly referred to as the eardrum, is the first obstruction in the canal and is a highly sensitive "drum skin," so to speak, which vibrates when stimulated by sound waves. When sound waves stimulate the tympanic membrane, the vibrations are neurologically transmitted to the brain for interpretation and response. It is the sensitivity of the eardrum that makes it vulnerable to attack, which results in excruciating pain.

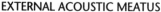

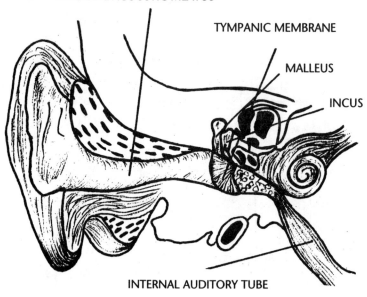

EXTERNAL ACOUSTIC MEATUS

TYMPANIC MEMBRANE

MALLEUS

INCUS

INTERNAL AUDITORY TUBE

FIGURE 47

Though the eardrum itself cannot be touched directly by anatomical weapons, a cupped hand slapped strongly over the ears will force air down the internal acoustic meatus, causing the eardrum to burst. Figure 48 is a head-on view of the middle ear and the eardrum. Immediately behind the middle ear is the inner ear—the most important area of the ear as a target.

Equilibrium is the ability to maintain balance. The part of the ear responsible for this function is the utricle, which is located in the inner ear. If the utricle is not functioning, you cannot walk or even stand without falling. The utricle detects where your head is in relation to your body position. When the ears are attacked effectively, the utricle temporarily ceases to send information to the brain. Based on information from such sensory organs and the peripheral nervous system, the brain acts to store and process information, then sends commands

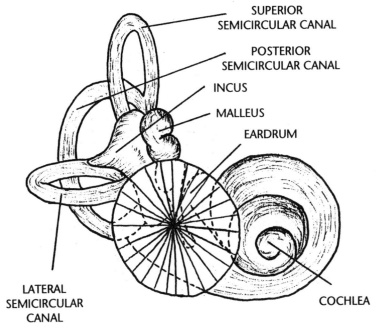

SUPERIOR
SEMICIRCULAR CANAL

POSTERIOR
SEMICIRCULAR CANAL

INCUS

MALLEUS

EARDRUM

LATERAL
SEMICIRCULAR
CANAL

COCHLEA

FIGURE 48

to the body to react to a given stimulus. Thus, when the utricle ceases to function, the brain does not know where the head is in relation to the rest of the body and, consequently, does not know which skeletal muscles to contract to maintain the body in an upright position. Balance cannot be maintained without this information. So when you attack the ears, you are attacking the nucleus of physical combat: balance. An effective attack to this area will not only cause excruciating pain, it will send an opponent to the ground without the physical ability to stand back up.

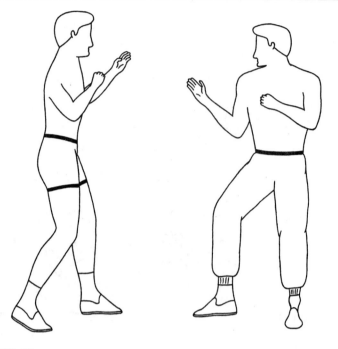

FIGURE 49

Practical Application Techniques #6 and #7

We are going to look at two techniques that target the ears, one with a block-and-strike movement and one in a grappling situation. You will want to keep in mind that, as with the eyes, the ears are prime targets in close-contact situations.

Technique #6 is illustrated in Figures 49 through 51. In Figure 49, your opponent is standing in a ready position, and you are in a flat-footed cat stance. Remember that your weight is supported entirely on the rear leg in this stance. In Figure 50, your opponent has stepped in with a wide left roundhouse punch. Lunge your body forward into a deep forward stance and meet the incoming punch with an inside suto block. As you do this, open your left hand for the return strike.

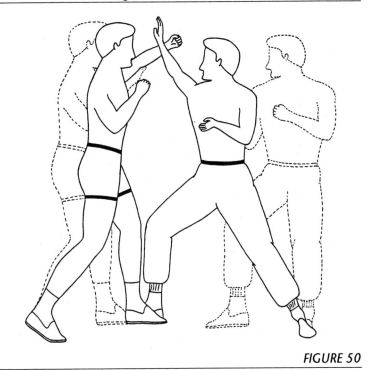

FIGURE 50

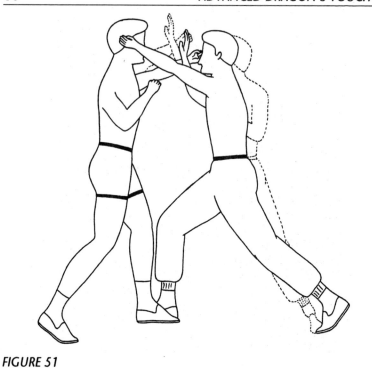

FIGURE 51

In a wide, sweeping motion utilizing centrifugal force (fig. 51), strike the opponent's right ear with your cupped left hand. In this hand position, be sure to press the fingers and the thumb together while keeping the fingers straight through the distal joints but slightly bent at the knuckles.

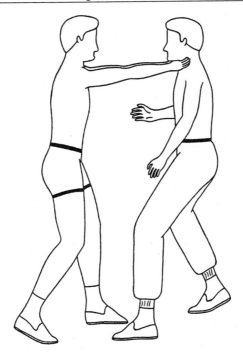

FIGURE 52

Technique #7 will start from a two-hand choke position (fig. 52). Note that the attacking arms are fully extended. If the arms were bent, the counterattack would be easier to execute because the targets would be closer. In Figures 53 and 54, you cup your hands as described in the previous technique and strike both ears simultaneously with as much force as you can generate.

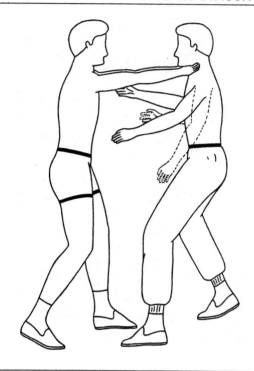

FIGURE 53

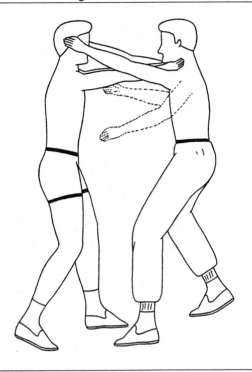

FIGURE 54

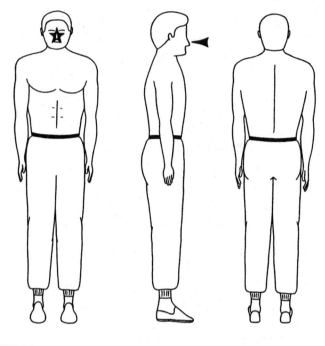

FIGURE 55

PRESSURE POINT #4: SEPTAL CARTILAGE

Observe Figure 55. The common term for the septal cartilage is the nose. It is the external portion of the respiratory system that partially protrudes from the face and acts as a filter for airborne foreign particles that become trapped in secreted mucosa and the nasal hairs that line the passages. The septal cartilage is firmly set in the nasal cavity of the skull (fig. 56), where the majority of its mass is hidden from view.

As its name indicates, it is a cartilaginous structure, not a bone as is commonly believed. Striking the septal cartilage on a horizontal plane usually ruptures the nasal portion of the angular vein and will cause tearing of the eyes and pain and, if it is a high-impact blow, will usually break it. The bleeding that accompanies a broken nose is generally profuse and somewhat difficult to

NASAL CAVITY

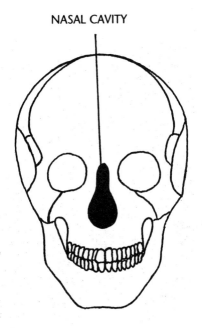

FIGURE 56

stop. Observe Figure 57. Typically the nose extends outward above the lower lip and protrudes from the face. An inclining blow at 45 degrees that strikes the nose at its bottom could easily send the nose upward through the christa galli and into the brain. Death would be instantaneous.

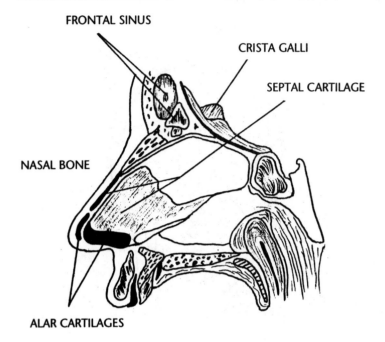

FRONTAL SINUS

CRISTA GALLI

SEPTAL CARTILAGE

NASAL BONE

ALAR CARTILAGES

FIGURE 57

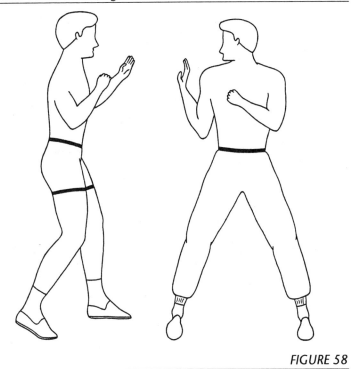

FIGURE 58

Practical Application Technique #8

You will be positioned in a right-faced straddle stance with your defensive arm (right) held as far to the rear as is comfortable (fig. 58). You are trying to draw a wide right punch to the face, so you want to give the appearance that the area is vulnerable to attack. As the punch begins to extend, block it away with a crossing palm block while leaning back slightly in your stance (fig. 59). Do not step back; lean back. This is a speed technique, so you will want to hold your stance. With a return lean, thrust your arm forward into your opponent's nose, striking with a chicken wrist (fig. 60).

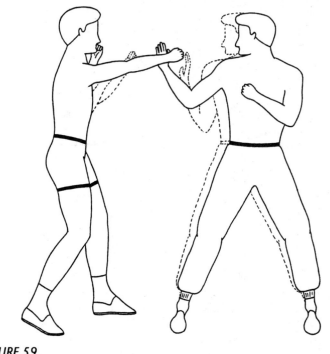

FIGURE 59

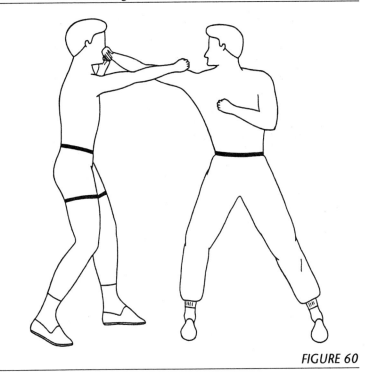

FIGURE 60

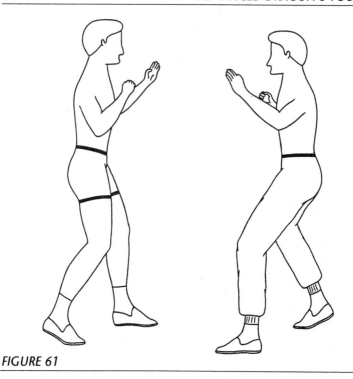

FIGURE 61

Practical Application Technique #9

Both you and your opponent begin in ready stances (fig. 61), and you will use a shuffle step in this technique with a short straight-line half-turn punch. In Figure 62, your opponent has lunged in to throw a right-handed face punch. The step is completed, and the punch is en route. In Figure 63, you take a slight step to the outside of the punch and use a crossing palm block with your left hand to carry the punch safely away from your face. Do not power the block into the movement. Bump the arm away just slightly so your counterblow will not be interfered with. With your right hand, you return a half-turn punch to your opponent's nose (fig. 64).

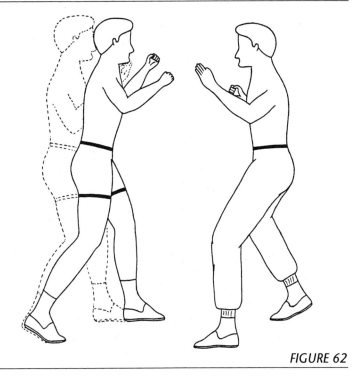

FIGURE 62

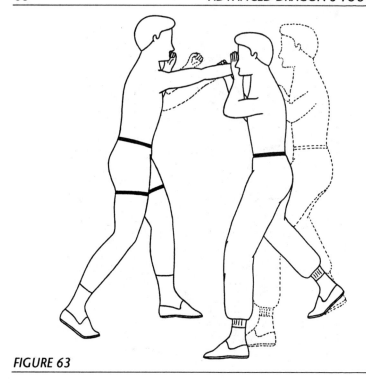

FIGURE 63

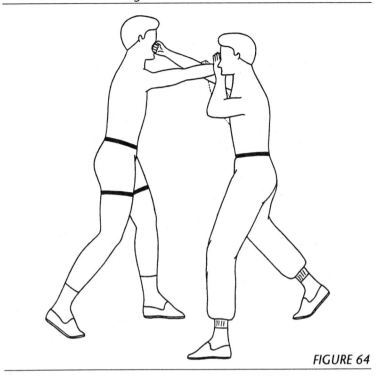

FIGURE 64

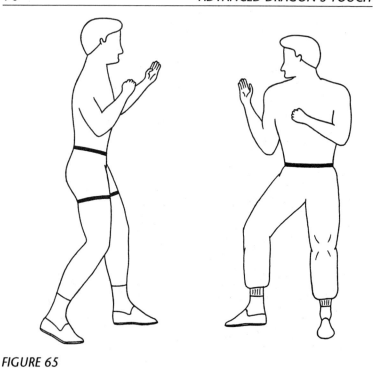

FIGURE 65

Practical Application Technique #10

Here you are positioned in a flat-footed cat stance (fig. 65). You are poised for quick movement, and this attack to the septal cartilage is designed to be lethal. In Figure 66, your opponent has initiated a wide left-hook punch at your face (these types of punches are typical in street fights). Your movement in Figure 67 is a forward lunge, with the lead hand formed for a palm strike directed at the nose. The arrow depicts the line of drive. The blow is not illustrated to full extension in order to show the amount of penetration that is achieved with this technique.

If this palm strike is properly powered and follows the line of drive shown, at the very least the blow will break the opponent's nose and send him sprawling backward to the floor. If the attack is perfect, the opponent will be killed instantly.

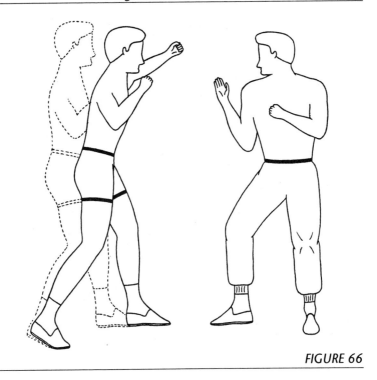

FIGURE 66

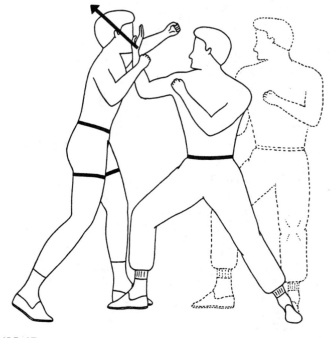

FIGURE 67

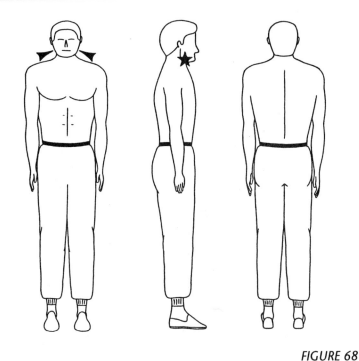

FIGURE 68

PRESSURE POINT #5: MANDIBLE

As a target, the mandible has three distinct points of contact designed to induce specific physiological responses. Two of these areas will be dealt with in this sequence; the third will be addressed separately with the next pressure point. You will note that two different target areas are shown in Figure 68. The center figure illustrates the jaw line below the hinge; the first figure denotes the hinge itself.

The mandible, which is shaded in Figure 69, is the only bone of the head over which there is muscular control—or which moves at all for that matter. All of the other bones above the cervical vertebrae are fused and fixed. The temporomandibular joint, which attaches the mandible to the skull, is a free-moving joint with two separate points of attachment on each side. The deep

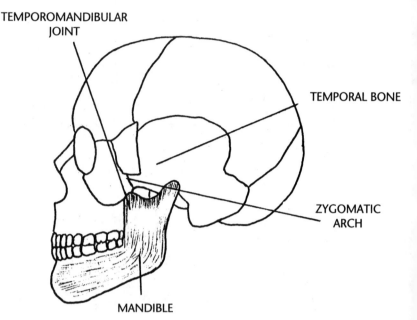

TEMPOROMANDIBULAR
JOINT

TEMPORAL BONE

ZYGOMATIC
ARCH

MANDIBLE

FIGURE 69

auricular branch of the internal maxillary artery, which
is usually ruptured when the hinge is broken, passes
through these articulations. A broken jaw is a painful
experience, both at the time of the injury and for several
weeks during the healing process. The mandible itself is
not easily broken, but enough force applied against the
mandible body compresses the joint and can break it.

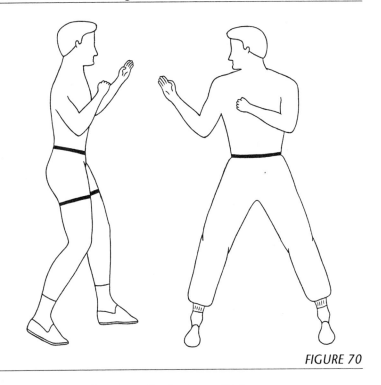

FIGURE 70

Practical Application Technique #11

Beginning from a right-faced straddle stance (fig. 70), you will again be using the fixed-stance defense, so you will want to set your legs to a depth that is both strong and comfortable. As your opponent advances with a straight punch to your face (fig. 71), raise your right arm and strike his arm above the wrist and continue the arc of movement till your blocking arm reaches the position at the end of the arrow. Your opponent's arm will be knocked down and out of your way by the block.

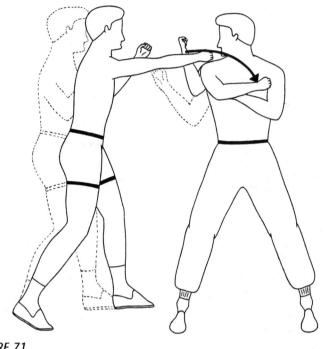

FIGURE 71

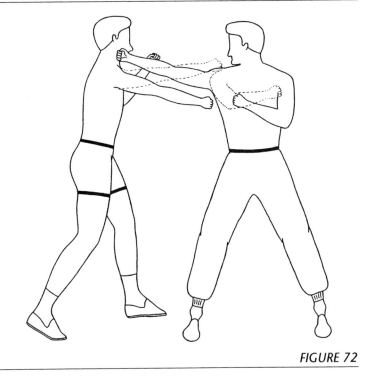

FIGURE 72

As in Figure 72, you immediately return a backhand strike to the curve of the mandible.

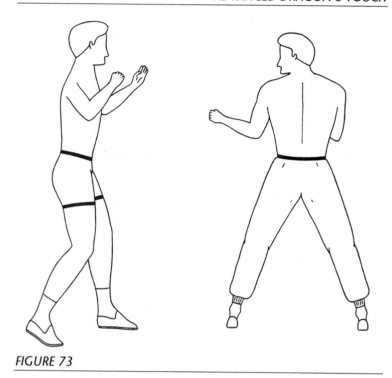

FIGURE 73

Practical Application Technique #12

In this sequence, you will be using a kick and initiating the first movement. This kick was studied in detail in *Da Qiang Ji: Power Striking.* Your starting position is a left-faced straddle stance (fig. 73), and this time you will be moving out of the stance. This entire movement is executed in a single flowing motion. The midpoint view in Figure 74 is a transient position showing the spinning hook kick in its chamber position. In Figure 75 you continue your spin and extend your kicking leg just as you reach the target. Strike with the back of your heel and continue your spin through the target.

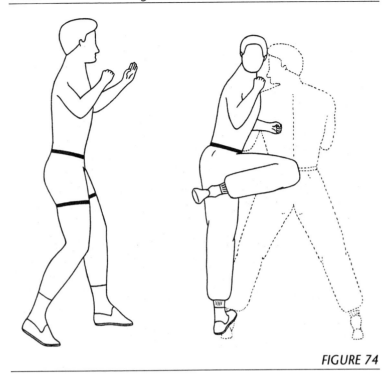

FIGURE 74

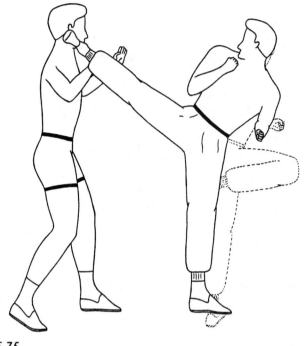

FIGURE 75

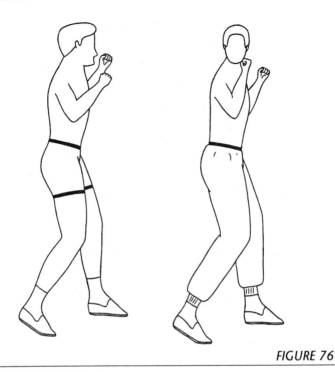

FIGURE 76

Practical Application Technique #13

In this final technique for the mandible, your opponent will be approaching from your rear, as in Figure 76. This is a combination technique using the lead strike as a setup. Look first at the step in the movement (fig. 77). This is a deep step and requires bending the stationary leg to allow the stepping foot to pass this far through and behind the lead foot. Snap out a high left backhand with just enough speed to conceal the fact that it is a setup blow and not intended to land. With optimum speed and power, spin your entire body to the right, striking your opponent on the mandible with a second backhand, as in Figure 78.

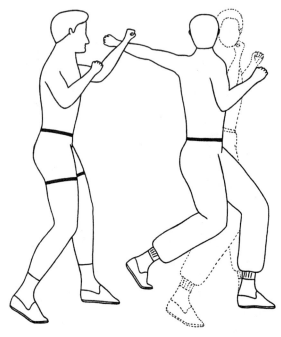

FIGURE 77

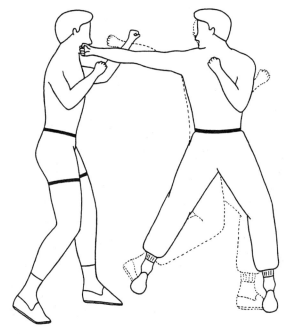

FIGURE 78

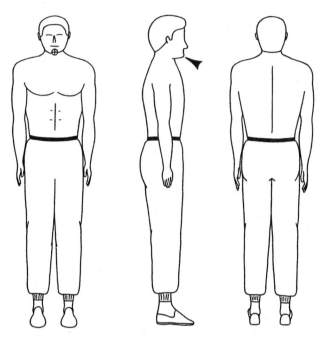

FIGURE 79

PRESSURE POINT #6: TIP OF THE MANDIBLE

The size of the opponent and the strength of his neck will have much to do with the amount of force required to accomplish the knockout this target is capable of yielding. Assuming there is moral justification for your engagement of the opponent, the recommended applied force is your absolute maximum. In Figure 79, the first and second illustrations depict your target area, with the arrow in the center showing the preferred direction of force. Observe Figures 80 and 81. These two skeletal illustrations denote your target area on the mandible, and Figure 81 illustrates how the rising stroke to the tip of the mandible results in what you might call a shock wave that passes through the rear of the skull.

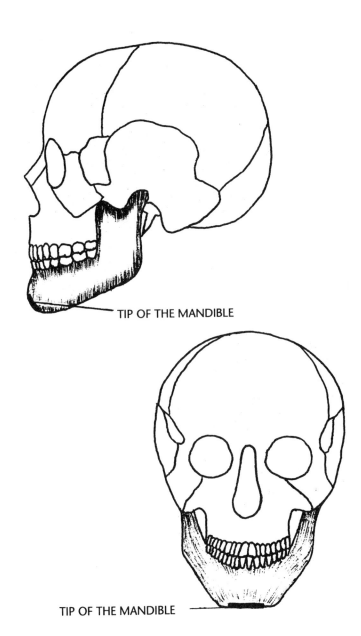

TIP OF THE MANDIBLE

TIP OF THE MANDIBLE

FIGURE 80

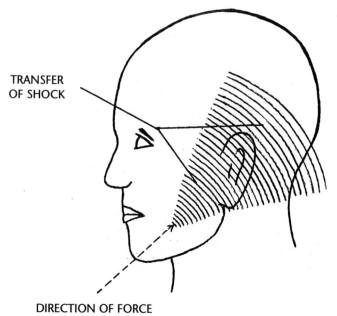

TRANSFER
OF SHOCK

DIRECTION OF FORCE

FIGURE 81

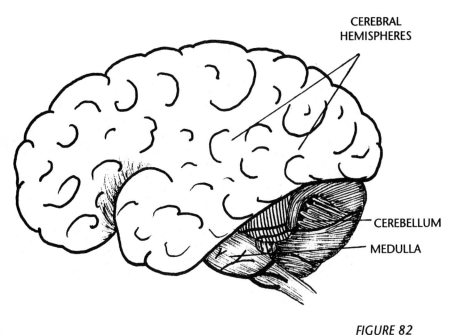

CEREBRAL
HEMISPHERES

CEREBELLUM

MEDULLA

FIGURE 82

Now look at Figure 82, and picture this illustration of the brain as it would appear inside the skull of Figure 81. When you look at the lines indicating the progression of the shock from the blow, and compare their location to Figure 82, you will see that the shock passes directly through the cerebral hemispheres. It is the shock to this area of the brain that causes the unconsciousness.

We're going to look at two practical application techniques for this pressure point: one using an elbow strike and one using a chicken wrist. Note that both of the blows impact on a rising plane to accomplish the cerebral jarring needed to effect a knockout.

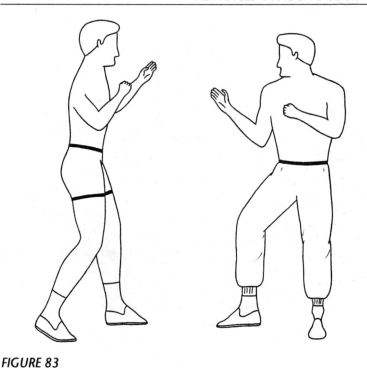

FIGURE 83

Practical Application Technique #14

In Figure 83, your opponent is in a ready stance, and you are positioned in a flat-footed cat stance. You will be using a block-and-wrap technique with a rising elbow return strike. As your opponent advances with a wide left punch (fig. 84), step outside his advancing foot and catch the incoming punch with an inside suto block. In Figure 85, you extend your arm over your opponent's arm, pull his arm into your armpit, and bring your elbow into your body, trapping his arm. His hand should be tucked into your armpit, and your hand should have a tight grip on his triceps. In a rising, crossing motion (fig. 86), strike the tip of your opponent's mandible with your left forearm.

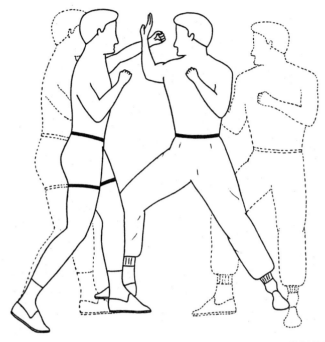

FIGURE 84

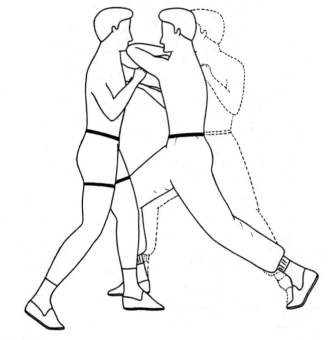

FIGURE 85

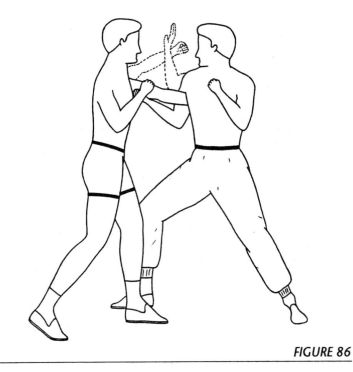

FIGURE 86

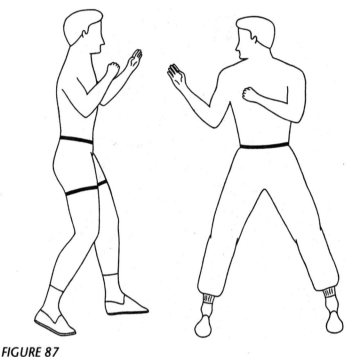

FIGURE 87

Practical Application Technique #15

Position yourself in a right-faced straddle stance, as in Figure 87. You will be taking a short rearward step in this technique. As your opponent advances with a straight right-hand punch (fig. 88), step across his stance and stop his incoming punch with a crossing palm block. Following the arrow in Figure 89, continue the flow of the blocking movement to the point illustrated. Finally, in a direct line following the needed incline (fig. 90), snap a chicken wrist blow up into the tip of your opponent's mandible.

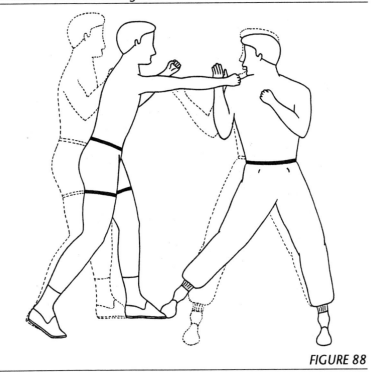

FIGURE 88

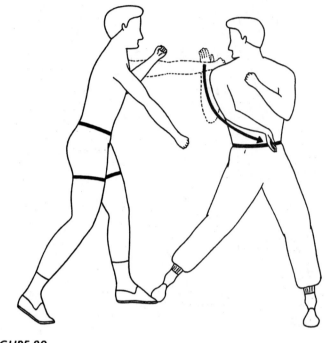

FIGURE 89

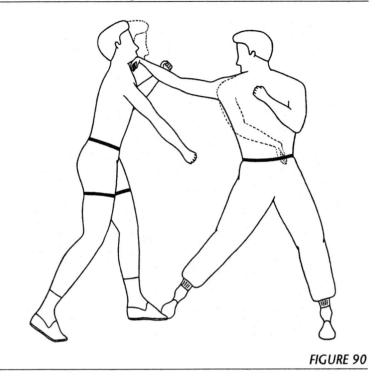

FIGURE 90

CHAPTER THREE

Pressure Points #7 through #10

The most conspicuous similarity between the four pressure points we will study in this chapter is that they are all located in the neck. The base of the cranium, pressure point #7, is in the back of the neck where it meets the skull; the cervical vertebrae, pressure point #9, is also in the back of the neck; the carotid plexus, pressure point #10, is located on both sides of the neck; and the anterior neck region, pressure point #8, is located in the front of the neck. The least conspicuous similarity between these pressure points is that they are all potentially lethal targets.

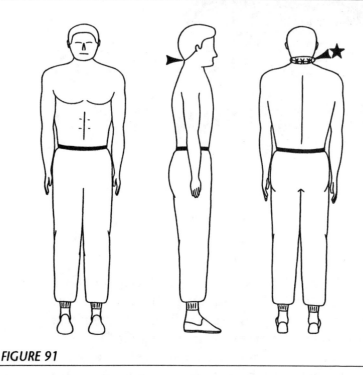

FIGURE 91

PRESSURE POINT #7: BASE OF THE CRANIUM

Observe Figure 91. The second and third illustrations depict the location of the target. The three Xs in the third figure indicate the points of contact more specifically, the center X being one target, while the two outside Xs pinpoint separate targets. As can be seen in Figure 92, the sternocliedomastoid muscle and part of the trapezius muscle attach at the base of the cranium at the point where the outside Xs are shown. A blow to this area generally causes unconsciousness. Figure 93 is a view of the cervical vertebrae as they meet the base of the cranium. This is the target denoted by the center X and is potentially lethal. (You will also want to look at Figure 119, pressure point #9, for another look at the cranial-vertebral junction.)

The first cervical vertebra is called the atlas. The cra-

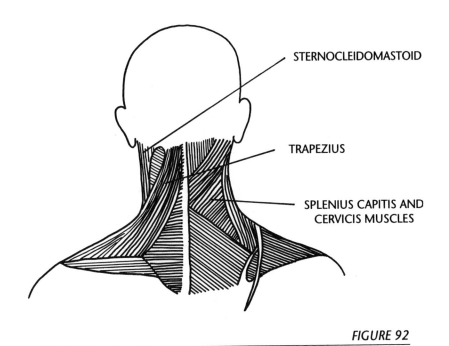

STERNOCLEIDOMASTOID

TRAPEZIUS

SPLENIUS CAPITIS AND
CERVICIS MUSCLES

FIGURE 92

nium does not rotate on this first vertebra; rather, it is fused to the skull and rotates on the second cervical vertebra, called the axis. The axis has a spindle that protrudes upward into it, providing a movable joint upon which the head is allowed basically free movement in all directions. If this joint was struck with sufficient force, the resulting damage would be total permanent paralysis below the head and would very probably be lethal if immediate medical attention was not available.

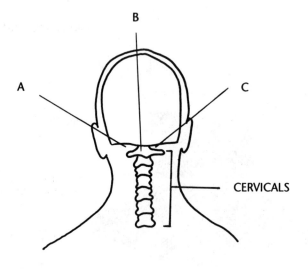

FIGURE 93

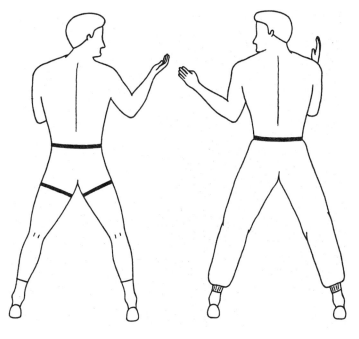

FIGURE 94

Practical Application Technique #16

Note the change in starting positions in Figure 94. Both you and your opponent are in side-faced straddle stances that do not oppose each other but rather face in the same direction. In Figure 95, your opponent has lunged forward to throw a long-reaching backhand. To reach the position depicted in Figure 96, take a slight step with your left foot as shown and rotate your right foot in a parallel direction. As your body is turning, block the incoming backhand with a left palm block. Turn your head fully to the right, bringing your opponent within the span of your peripheral vision. As in Figure 97, bring your right foot all the way around while pivoting on your left foot, and deliver a rearward vertical elbow to the base of your opponent's cranium.

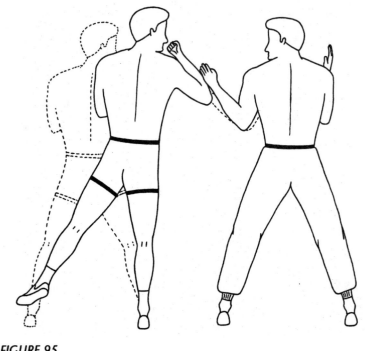

FIGURE 95

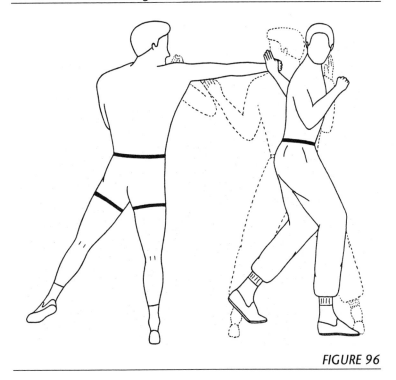

FIGURE 96

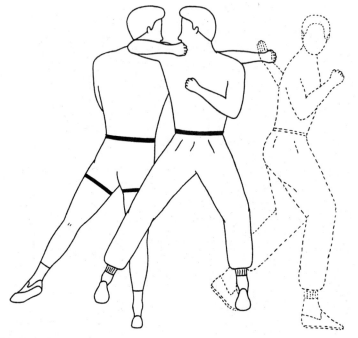

FIGURE 97

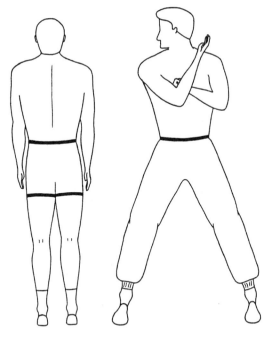

FIGURE 98

Practical Application Technique #17

This blow can be directed to the center target point or to the outside areas. Figure 98 shows the palm-down suto fully chambered; Figure 99 shows the blow extended into the target.

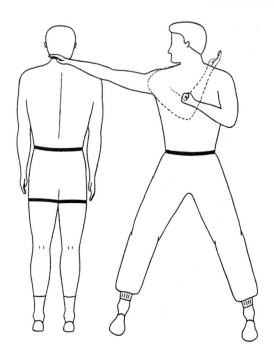

FIGURE 99

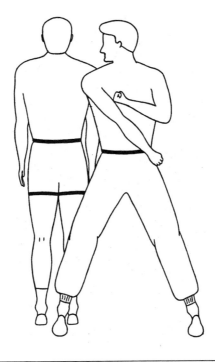

FIGURE 100

Practical Application Technique #18

This blow is similar to the counterattack illustrated in Technique #16, but here the elbow is delivered on a rising plane (figs. 100 and 101).

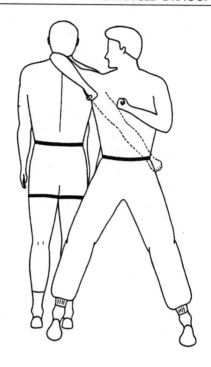

FIGURE 101

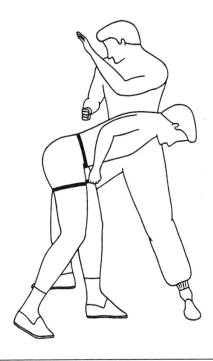

FIGURE 102

Practical Application Technique #19

Figures 102 and 103 illustrate a downward vertical elbow delivered at an angle to either of the target areas. It is not unusual to find yourself in such a position in the course of a physical confrontation. In this application the opponent is close to you. If he was farther away from you, the same stroke could be applied with a short step.

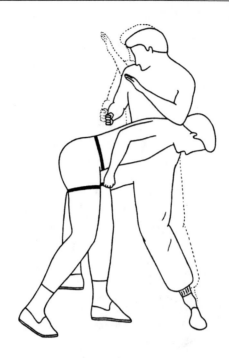

FIGURE 103

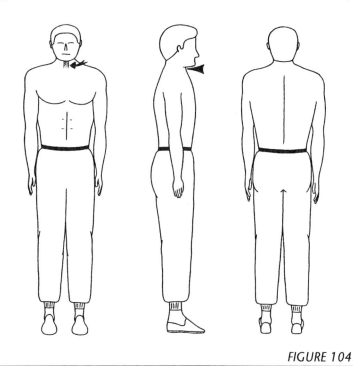

FIGURE 104

PRESSURE POINT #8: ANTERIOR NECK REGION

The anterior neck region is one of the most lethal targets in the human anatomy. Its life-sustaining structures are virtually unprotected and are sensitive to even low-impact blows. Figure 104 shows your target area. Figure 105 shows a cut-away view of the anterior neck region from the side. Locate the larynx and the trachea, and look at Figure 106. This is the area through which air is taken into the lungs. The larynx works with other communicating organs to prevent solids or liquids from entering the lungs via the trachea. The trachea itself is a flexible tube held in a cylindrical configuration by tiny C-shaped cartilages that prevent it from collapsing during inhalation. Figure 107 shows the esophagus, the tube leading into the stomach.

The functions of the organs in the anterior neck

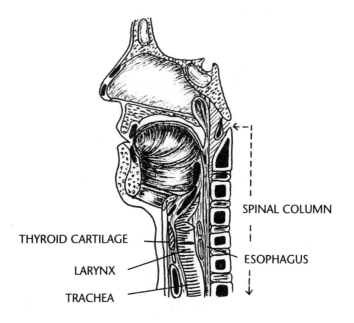

SPINAL COLUMN

THYROID CARTILAGE

LARYNX

TRACHEA

ESOPHAGUS

FIGURE 105

region are vital to life. Striking this area with a blow powerful enough to result in damage to the larynx, trachea, or thyroid cartilage could be lethal. The passage of air into the lungs would be prevented, resulting in asphyxiation, and the cartilages of the trachea would puncture the trachea tube or other organs in the area, causing blood to enter the lungs and resulting in drowning. Because these structures are protected only by a layer of skin, their vulnerability is apparent.

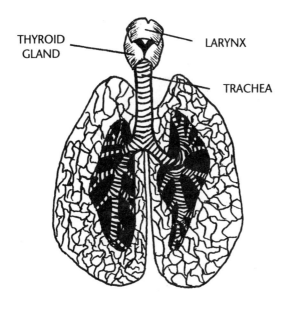

THYROID GLAND

LARYNX

TRACHEA

FIGURE 106

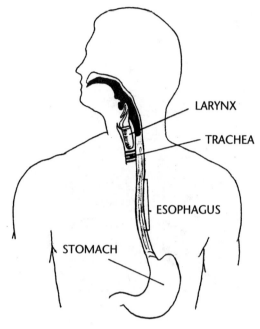

FIGURE 107

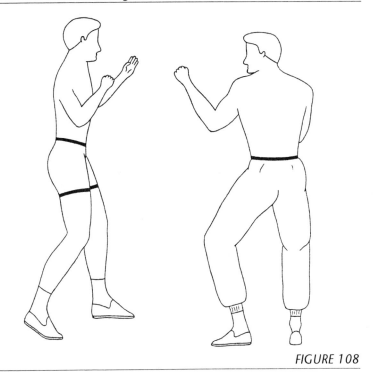

FIGURE 108

Practical Application Technique #20

In Figure 108, your opponent is in a ready stance, and you are in a close-legged back stance. In Figure 109, your opponent has advanced with a straight right hand. Shift your weight entirely onto your rear leg and chamber a left side kick. As you shift your weight, stop the progress of the incoming punch with an inside suto block. Then, with a pivot on the standing foot, extend your side kick into your opponent's anterior neck region (fig. 110).

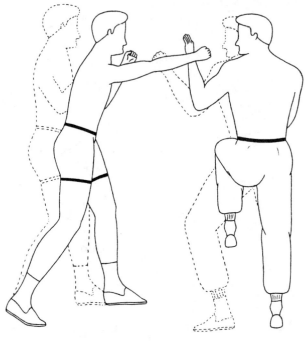

FIGURE 109

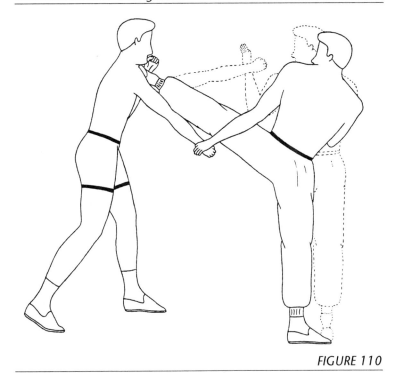

FIGURE 110

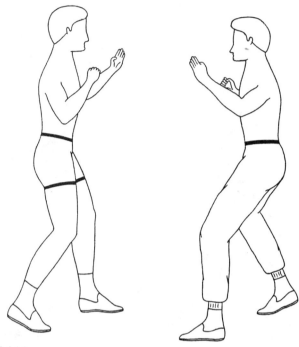

FIGURE 111

Practical Application Technique #21

In Figure 111, both you and your opponent are positioned in a ready stance. You will be countering with a short straight-line stroke designed for speed, utilizing the simultaneous block-and-strike principle. In Figure 112, your opponent has taken his advancing step, and his right-hand punch is en route. With a short outside step, guide the punch away from your face with a crossing palm block, as in Figure 113, and deliver a simultaneous forefist strike to your opponent's anterior neck region.

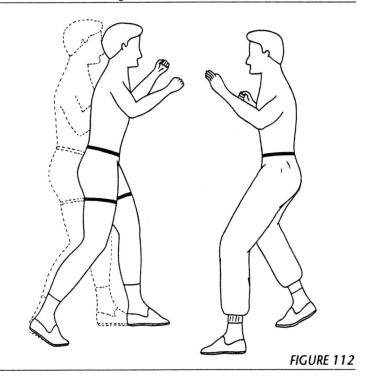

FIGURE 112

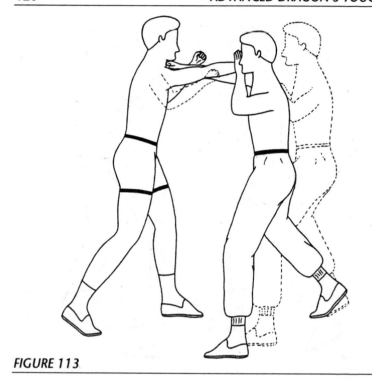

FIGURE 113

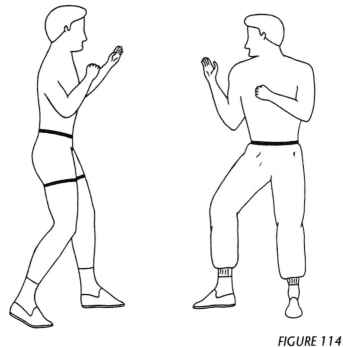

FIGURE 114

Practical Application Technique #22

In Figure 114 you are in a flat-footed cat stance, and your opponent is in a ready stance. Note that your lead hand is being held low and close to your body. You are trying to draw a left-hand punch to the face. As your opponent advances with a wide left hook (fig. 115), lunge to the outside of his lead foot into a forward stance and stop the incoming punch with a wide suto block. As in Figure 116, rotate your blocking hand, taking a grip on your opponent's arm, and drive a hook strike to your opponent's anterior neck region.

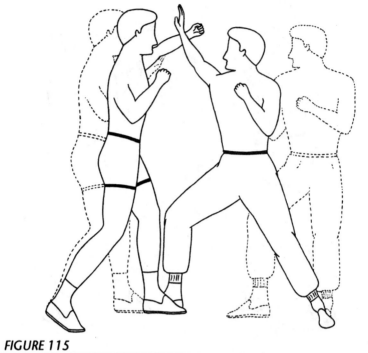

FIGURE 115

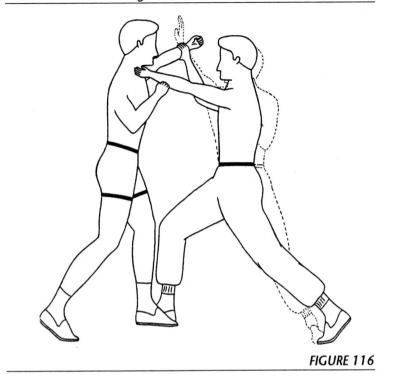

FIGURE 116

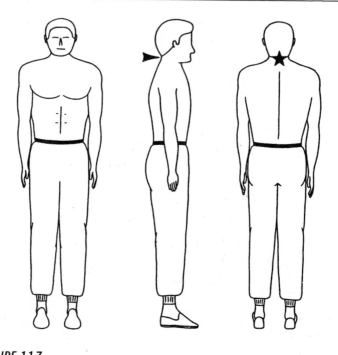

FIGURE 117

PRESSURE POINT #9: CERVICAL VERTEBRAE

Observe Figure 117. The cervical vertebrae extend from the base of the skull into the shoulders. Observe Figure 118. The first seven vertebrae beneath the skull are the cervicals. The eighth is the first of the thoracic group and is readily identified by the attachment of the first rib. The first seven vertebrae are our area of study here. As do all parts of the human anatomy, vertebrae serve a specific purpose. In addition to providing axial support and attachment for the skeletal structure, vertebrae provide a protective housing for the path of the spinal cord that supplies neural communication throughout the body from the brain. If any section of the spinal cord was severed, movement beneath the point of severance would no longer be possible. Because the neck is so high on the vertebral chain,

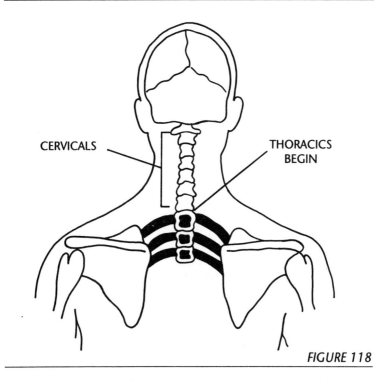

CERVICALS

THORACICS
BEGIN

FIGURE 118

damage to the spinal cord would leave the victim paralyzed below the neck and would likely be lethal if the damage occurred above the brachial plexus.

Figure 119 is an enlarged illustration of the cervical spine showing Group A and Group B. Emerging from Group A are the phrenic nerves, which maintain communication between the brain and diaphragm. The diaphragm is the voluntary/involuntary muscle that controls breathing. If it was "disconnected" from the brain by damage above the fifth cervical vertebra, respiratory paralysis would occur, resulting in asphyxiation. Therefore, strikes directed to the middle to upper area of the cervical spine are potentially lethal. Strikes to the lower portion of this target could be permanently debilitating.

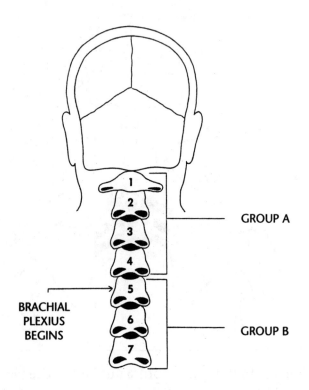

FIGURE 119

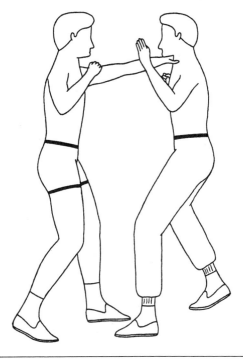

FIGURE 120

Practical Application Technique #23

In this attack, your opponent has grabbed you by the throat and drawn back his right hand for a punch (fig. 120). With your left hand, you catch the incoming punch with an inside suto block, as in Figure 121, while delivering a simultaneous half-turn punch to your opponent's chin. The purpose of the punch is to distract your opponent while getting your second arm inside both of his for your next move. His grip on your neck will be weakened from the punch. Bump the choking arm from your path and step forward. Place your right hand on your opponent's chin and your left hand on the top rear of his head, as in Figure 122. Pull your left hand down to your left side while holding your opponent's head firmly (fig. 123), and drive his chin upward with your right hand. This is a lethal technique.

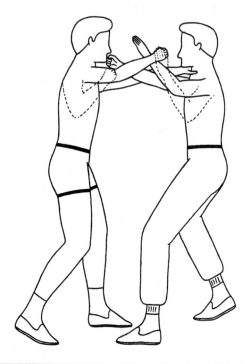

FIGURE 121

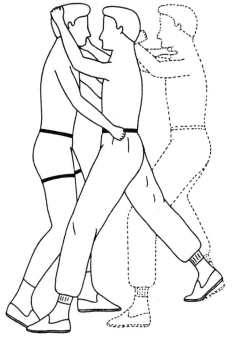

FIGURE 122

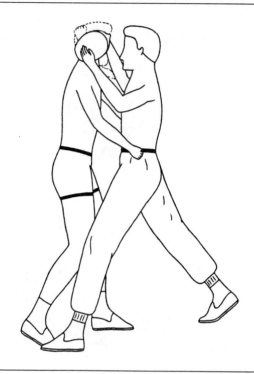

FIGURE 123

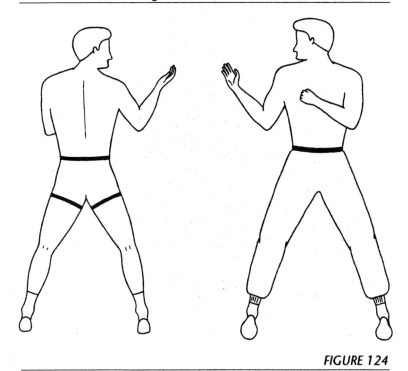

FIGURE 124

Practical Application Technique #24

In Figure 124, both you and your opponent are positioned in right-faced straddle stances, and you will be using a technique that utilizes a diversionary movement. With a forward hop, advance on your opponent and chamber your right leg for a low front kick (fig. 125). As in Figure 126, feint a low front kick at your opponent to draw his lead hand downward to block the kick. As you do this, chamber a crossing palm-down suto. In Figure 127, you set your right foot down, resuming your side straddle stance, and deliver a palm-down suto to your opponent's cervical vertebrae.

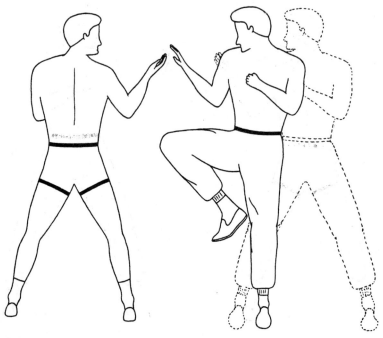

FIGURE 125

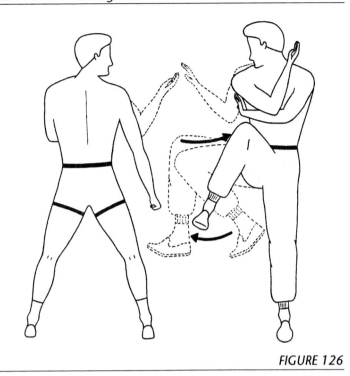

FIGURE 126

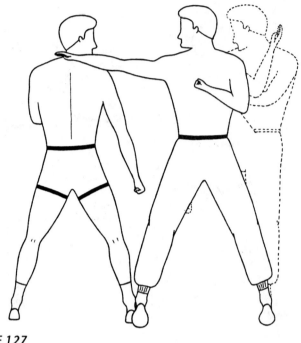

FIGURE 127

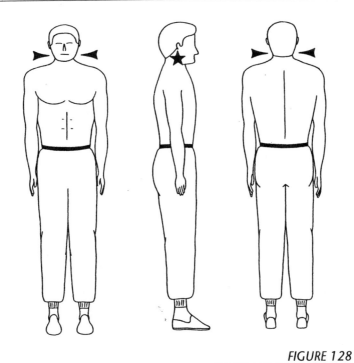

FIGURE 128

PRESSURE POINT #10: CAROTID PLEXUS

Look at Figures 128 and 129, then locate the denoted area on your own neck. Using a stiff index finger, poke this area with medium pressure. Striking this very sensitive area with high-impact blows will cause excruciating pain. The sternocliedomastoid muscle (fig. 130) is the superficial target and is one of the muscles that control the movement of the head. As depicted in the illustration, the muscle attaches at the clavicle and sterno-clavicle joint at the bottom and to the temporal bone at the mastoid at the top.

The extreme sensitivity of this muscle makes it a preferred target that can yield a variety of physiological responses ranging from unconsciousness to debilitating pain. Directly beneath this muscle is our actual target, the carotid plexus (figs. 131 and 132). In Figure 131, the

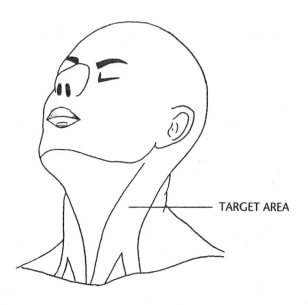

TARGET AREA

FIGURE 129

sternocliedomastoid muscle is pulled back to reveal the common carotid artery and the internal jugular vein. These two blood passages are the carotid plexus, responsible for the arterial feed and the venous return of blood between the heart and the brain. Figure 132 is an illustration of the carotid plexus outside its position in the neck. When you interrupt the flow of blood to and from the brain, you cause unconsciousness. If the interruption is substantial and sustained, brain damage is probable and death likely. A blow to this area with enough force to damage either blood tract will be lethal if immediate medical attention is not available.

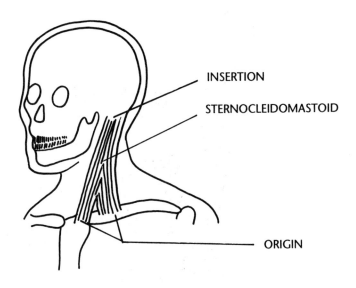

INSERTION

STERNOCLEIDOMASTOID

ORIGIN

FIGURE 130

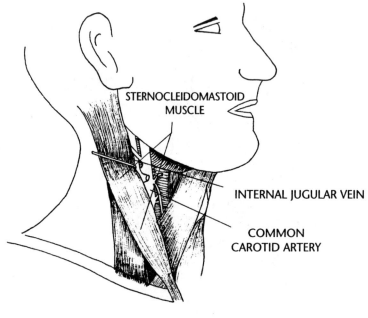

STERNOCLEIDOMASTOID
MUSCLE

INTERNAL JUGULAR VEIN

COMMON
CAROTID ARTERY

FIGURE 131

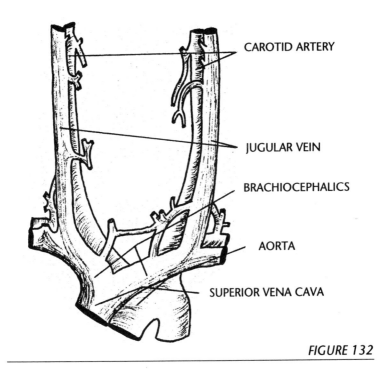

CAROTID ARTERY

JUGULAR VEIN

BRACHIOCEPHALICS

AORTA

SUPERIOR VENA CAVA

FIGURE 132

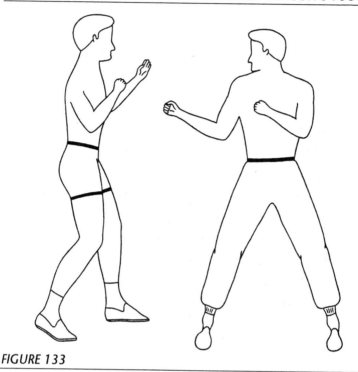

FIGURE 133

Practical Application Technique #25

You will begin in a side-faced straddle stance (fig. 133), and your opponent will be in a ready position. Look closely at Figures 134 through 137; this counter-attack will be from a combination punch. In Figure 134, your opponent has advanced with a left half-turn punch at your face. Lean back slightly in your stance and block the incoming punch with a right inside suto block. In Figure 135, your opponent advances again, this time with a double shuffle step, and throws a right-hand punch. Pivot all the way around on your left foot, turning to your right, and palm grab the incoming punch on the outside. At the completion of your movement you will be in a left-faced, close-legged cat stance. As in Figures 136 and 137, chamber a left roundhouse kick, then release the kick while pivoting on your standing foot.

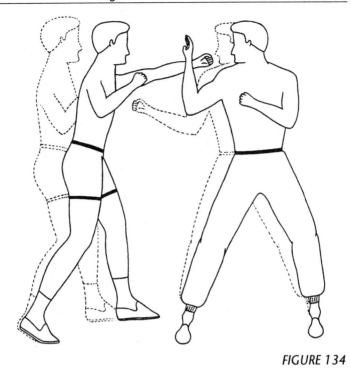

FIGURE 134

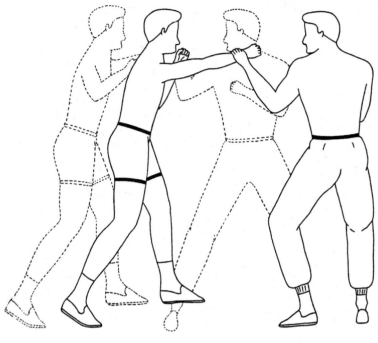

FIGURE 135

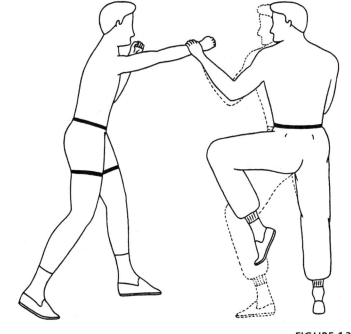

FIGURE 136

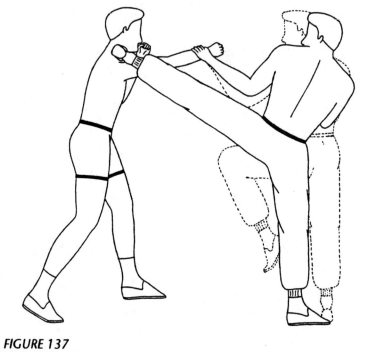

FIGURE 137

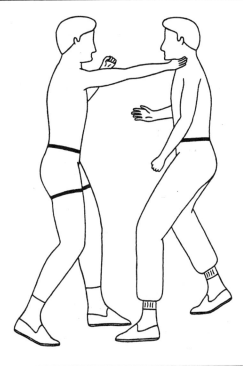

FIGURE 138

Practical Application Technique #26

In this sequence you will begin from a one-handed choke attack (fig. 138) and will counter with a break-away block and a return stroke. In Figure 139, you bring your right foot forward to prepare for a coming step and raise your right arm for the breakaway block. Pivoting on the right foot (fig. 140), step back with the left into a straddle stance while breaking off the choke with a crossing stroke of the right arm. Now return a palm-down suto to your opponent's carotid plexus (fig. 141).

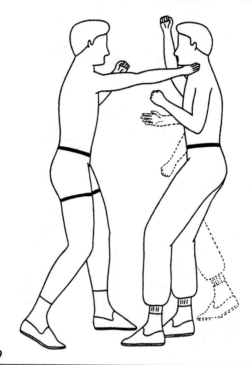

FIGURE 139

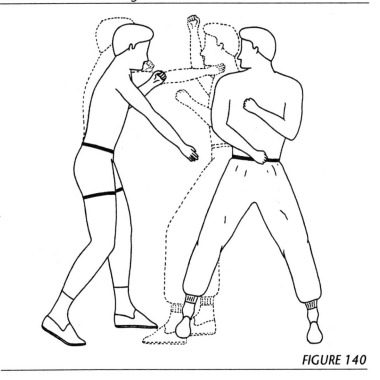

FIGURE 140

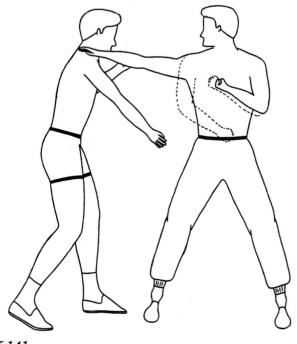

FIGURE 141

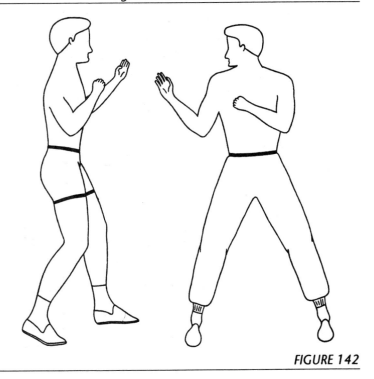

FIGURE 142

Practical Application Technique #27

In this technique, you begin in a side-faced straddle stance, while your opponent is in a ready position (fig. 142). As your opponent takes a forward step to release a right hand (fig. 143), step slightly to your rear, placing your right foot just outside his advancing foot. Prepare for a down-stroke palm block by raising your right hand slightly. With a crossing circular motion, strike the incoming punch downward and continue the flow of the stroke to the position shown in Figure 144. As you do this, rotate your stance and chamber a wide inside suto. Using an additional rotation to enhance your impact power, strike your opponent's carotid plexus with a left inside suto, as in Figure 145.

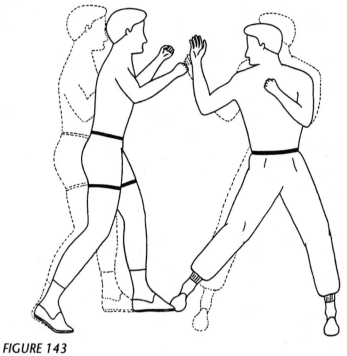

FIGURE 143

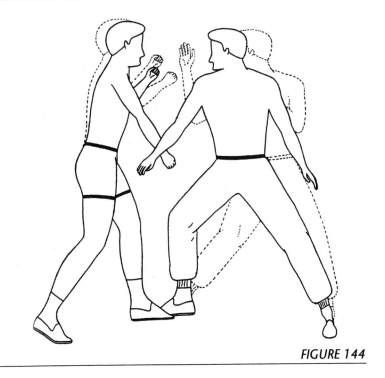

FIGURE 144

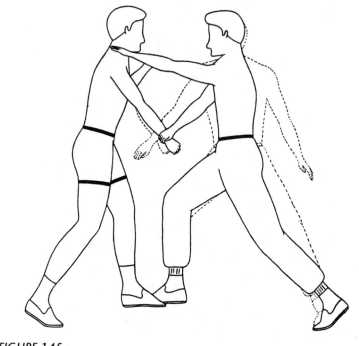

FIGURE 145

CHAPTER FOUR

Pressure Points #11 through #15

Of the five pressure points we will cover in this chapter, three are neuromuscular knockout points and two are skeletostructural attacks. Two of the points are potentially lethal, depending upon the physical condition of the opponent and the rate of force applied to the target. Pressure point #11 is the brachial plexus, #12 is the suprasternal notch, #13 is the heart, #14 is the sternum, and #15 is the solar plexus. These targets are located from the top of the shoulders to the top of the abdomen.

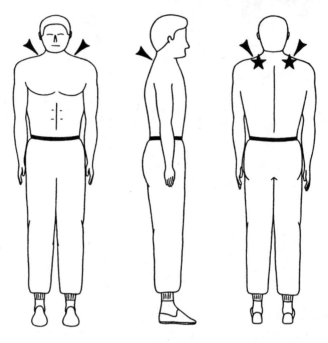

FIGURE 146

PRESSURE POINT #11: BRACHIAL PLEXUS

The brachial plexus is a complex interweaving of nerves originating from five pairs of nerve roots that descend from three of the cervical vertebrae and two of the thoracic vertebrae. Figure 146 depicts the surface point of attack for this pressure point. Figure 147 depicts the origin and descent of the brachial plexus. Figures 148 and 149 depict the trapezius muscle, which acts largely as a protective covering for this plexus, in addition to its function as skeletal muscle.

A strike to the brachial plexus at the point denoted by the stars in Figure 146 will result in a knockout. The brachial plexus may also be compressed by striking the trapezius muscle—visible from the facing side of the body—over the shoulders, but because the contact is less direct, this technique is also less likely to cause uncon-

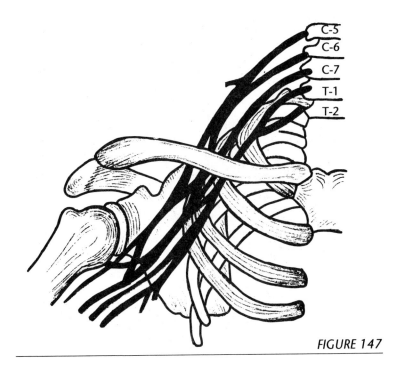

C-5
C-6
C-7
T-1
T-2

FIGURE 147

sciousness. The most likely result of an attack at this angle is the temporary paralysis of the corresponding arm. The majority of the neural communication between the brain and the arm occurs through the brachial plexus, and sufficiently powered blows to this area will paralyze the arm temporarily.

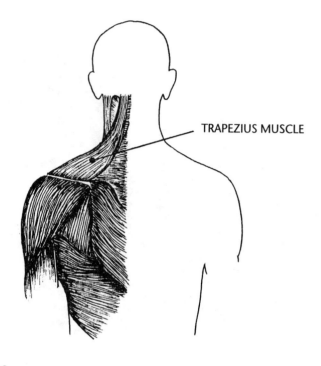

TRAPEZIUS MUSCLE

FIGURE 148

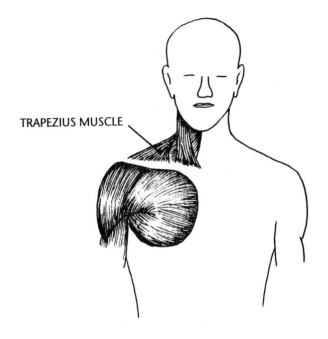

TRAPEZIUS MUSCLE

FIGURE 149

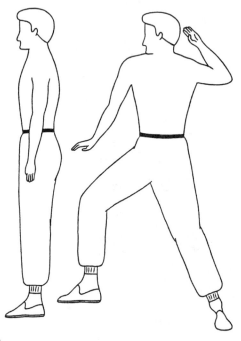

FIGURE 150

Practical Application Technique #28

The most direct, effective attack to the brachial plexus comes from a rear approach, as depicted in Figures 150 and 151. Note the differences in both the upper and lower body from the chamber position depicted in Figure 150 and the delivery position depicted in Figure 151. Compound power movements were discussed in detail in *Da Qiang Ji: Power Striking*, and those power systems applied with this technique will produce a guaranteed knockout.

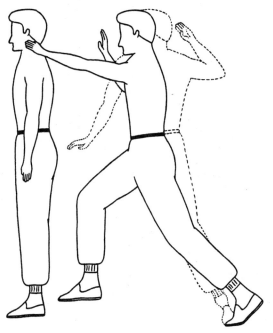

FIGURE 151

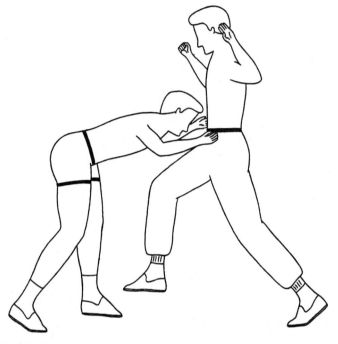

FIGURE 152

Practical Application Technique #29

Figures 152 and 153 depict what is a common position to find yourself in during a street confrontation—that of your opponent attempting to tackle you. Again, you have used a vertical suto to the brachial plexus (although once your opponent has grabbed you, a vertical elbow stroke would be more practical because the target would be closer).

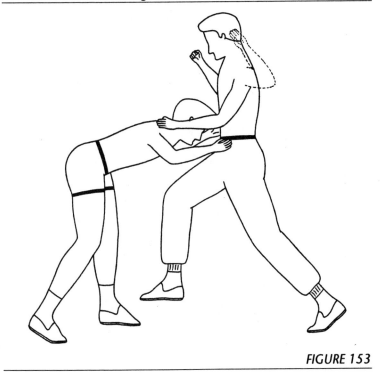

FIGURE 153

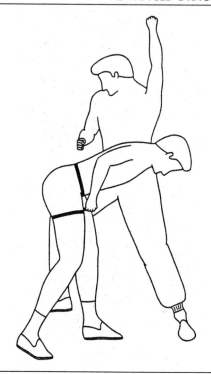

FIGURE 154

Practical Application Technique #30

In Figures 154 and 155, you are again in close proximity to your opponent, who is bent over at the waist. This vertical elbow stroke is directed to the brachial plexus and may be followed by a rising knee to the sternum or face with only a minor shift in your standing position.

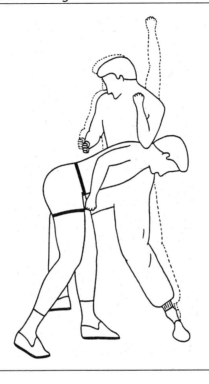

FIGURE 155

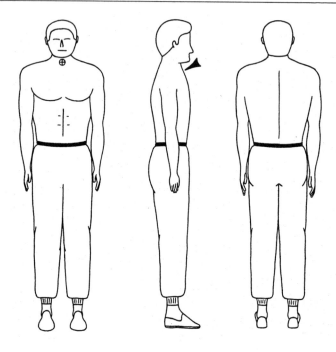

FIGURE 156

PRESSURE POINT #12: SUPRASTERNAL NOTCH

The anatomical term "suprasternal notch" describes the depression at the junction of the clavicles (collarbones) and the sternum. In Figure 156, the target area is shown in the first and second figures. Look also at Figure 157, which is a detailed illustration of the clavicles as they meet the sternum. The clavicles are made of bone, and the sternum is made of cartilage. There is a slight depression at the top end of the sternum, which is easily felt by the index finger.

Now look at Figure 158 and review pressure point #10, the carotid plexus, and Figure 132. The superior vena cava and the aorta are the main blood tracts that connect the carotid plexus to the heart, and these tracts lie just beneath the suprasternal notch. You will also recall having studied pressure point #8, the anterior

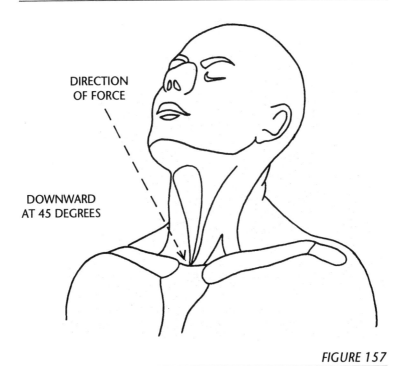

DIRECTION
OF FORCE

DOWNWARD
AT 45 DEGREES

FIGURE 157

neck region, and Figure 107, showing how the trachea passes beneath the suprasternal notch. This pressure point is most vulnerable at the junction of the clavicles. A high-impact blow to this area can dislodge the clavicles from the sternum. The loose bones could rupture the aorta, the superior vena cava, or the trachea, all of which are potentially lethal injuries.

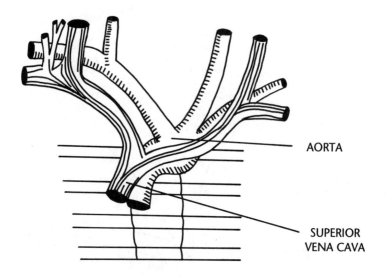

AORTA

SUPERIOR
VENA CAVA

FIGURE 158

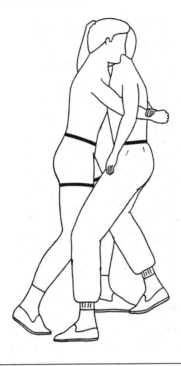

FIGURE 159

Practical Application Technique #31

Your starting position (fig. 159) is from a front bear hug under the arms. Your first movement is to get a good grip on your opponent's hair at the area shown. Do not pull the head back; jerk it back sharply, as in Figure 160, and chamber a downward vertical elbow strike with your opposite arm. As in Figure 161, drive your downward vertical elbow stroke into your opponent's suprasternal notch.

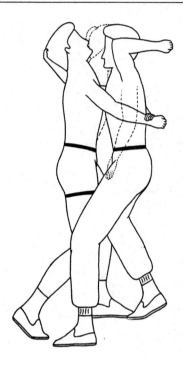

FIGURE 160

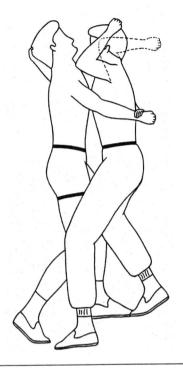

FIGURE 161

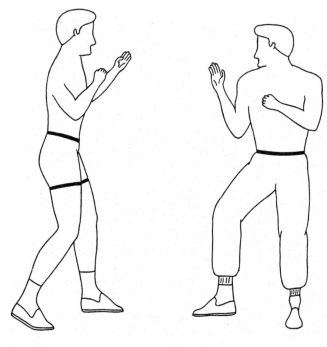

FIGURE 162

Practical Application Technique #32

The block-and-return technique you and your opponent are set up for in Figure 162 requires expert execution, especially in the delivery of the block. Pay close attention to the arm positions and the accompanying instructions with each frame.

As your opponent steps forward with a vertical jab (fig. 163), step outside the incoming punch and slightly forward. When you deliver this double outside hammer block, the movement of the left arm is only a slight bump on the incoming arm; the movement at the right arm is a full-power strike to the lower triceps (back arm muscle) just above the elbow, using the blocking area of the arm as a striking weapon. Now lean back slightly while chambering a high left hammer strike (fig. 164), and continue the motion of your right arm by following a half-circular motion counterclockwise. Finally, rotate

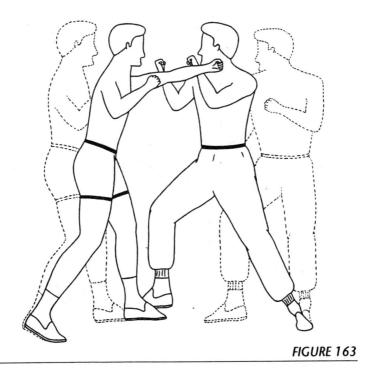

FIGURE 163

your entire body toward your opponent and deliver a left hammer strike to your opponent's suprasternal notch, as in Figure 165.

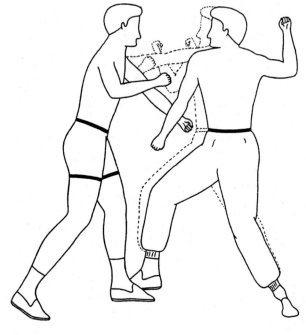

FIGURE 164

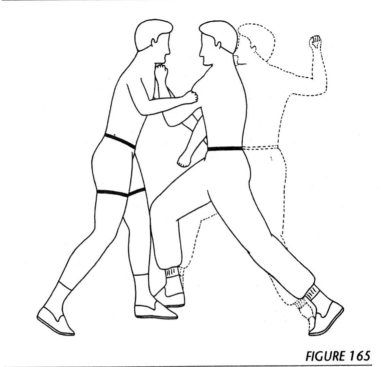

FIGURE 165

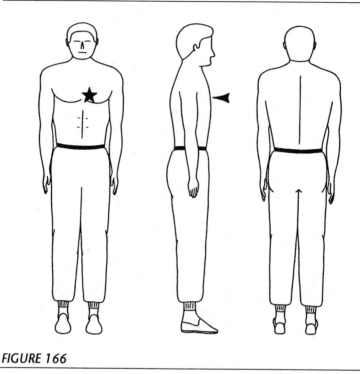

FIGURE 166

PRESSURE POINT #13: THE HEART

The structural design of the thorax provides a cage around the heart and lungs to protect these sensitive life-supporting organs. Because of this protective structure, the heart cannot be hit directly by conventional anatomical weapons. However, blows designed and delivered to produce a concussion effect can shock the heart, and deep-driving high-impact blows can have a similar effect. The age and physical condition of an opponent will also have a bearing on the outcome of attacks to the heart. The more out of shape and the older the opponent, the more susceptible his heart will be to technical attacks.

Observe Figure 166. Note that the target area is not directly along the centerline. Now observe Figures 167, 168, and 169. Note that though the centerline does pass

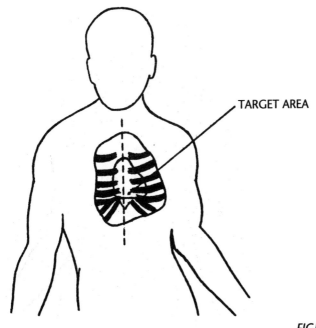

TARGET AREA

FIGURE 167

through the heart, the bulk of its mass lies to the left. For this reason, you will want to direct your attacks to the heart to the left of the centerline, as denoted in Figures 166 and 168.

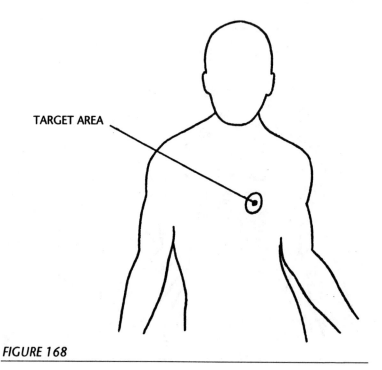

TARGET AREA

FIGURE 168

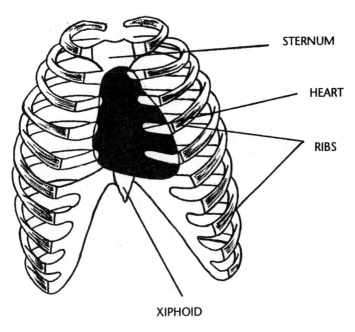

STERNUM

HEART

RIBS

XIPHOID

FIGURE 169

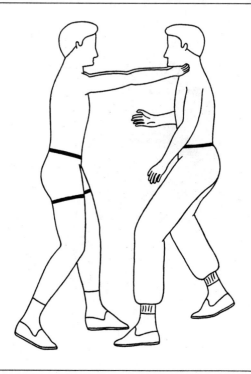

FIGURE 170

Practical Application Technique #33

In Figure 170, your opponent has you in a front two-handed choke, arms extended. Begin by reaching over your opponent's arms and using your left hand as a hook (fig. 171), and then bend the corresponding wrist and exert a crossing downward pull to hold him in position for your counterstrike. Now, with maximum speed and power, fire a vertical concussion punch into your opponent's heart (fig. 172). Remember that the concussion punch stops with one inch of penetration. It is the shock that follows the flow of the movement that passes through the heart.

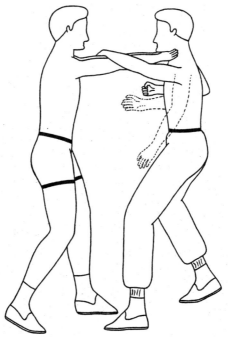

FIGURE 171

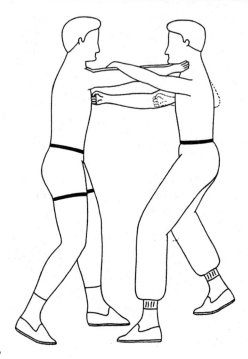

FIGURE 172

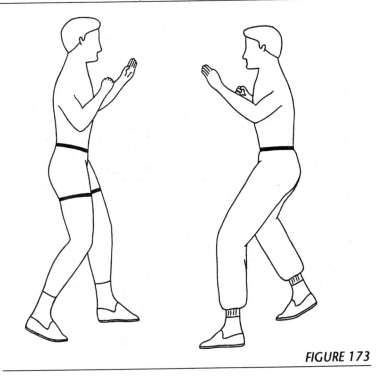

FIGURE 173

Practical Application Technique #34

Starting from ready positions (fig. 173), you will be using an outside slip movement and a fully powered centrifugal force counterstrike. As your opponent advances with a straight right hand, take a slightly forward and outside step and chamber a wide horizontal palm strike (fig. 174). As in Figure 175, drive your horizontal palm strike into your opponent's heart.

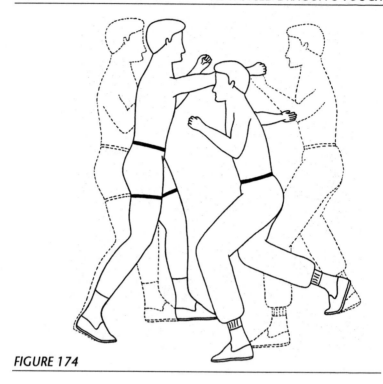

FIGURE 174

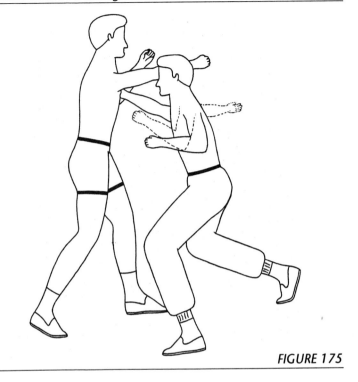

FIGURE 175

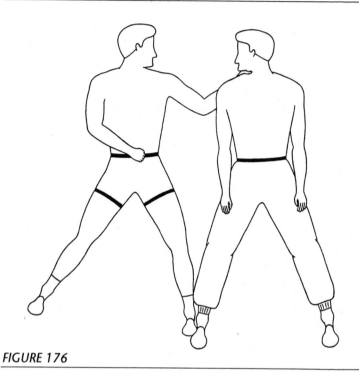

FIGURE 176

Practical Application Technique #35

In your starting position (fig. 176), your opponent
has approached you from your right side and grabbed
you with a one-handed choke. As in Figure 177, raise
your arms to the low chamber position for a right backhand. Now refer back to Chapter 1, Figures 17 and 18.
The Figure 17 posture focuses on the first two knuckles;
Figure 18 concentrates on the flat top of the hand,
which is used to apply concussion motion penetration
to larger areas. When you deliver the backhand shown
in Figure 178, use the Figure 18 posture with the one-
inch concussion penetration motion.

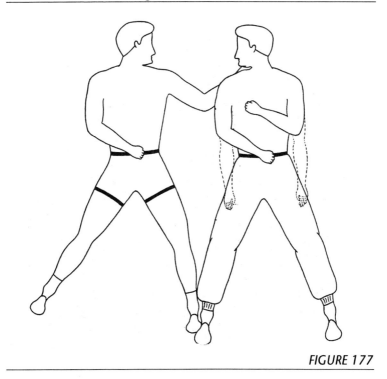

FIGURE 177

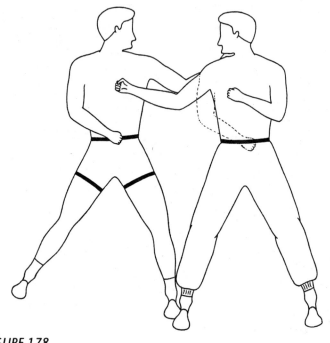

FIGURE 178

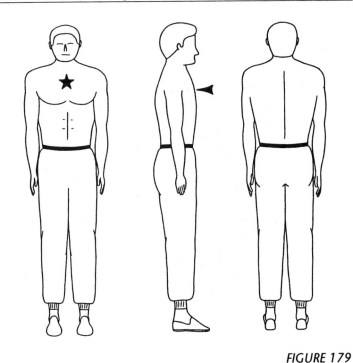

FIGURE 179

PRESSURE POINT #14: STERNUM

Observe Figure 179. The sternum, sometimes called the breastbone, is the narrow solid area between the pectoralis muscles that runs from the suprasternal notch (pressure point #12) to the solar plexus (pressure point #15) at the top of the abdominal muscles. It is constructed of cartilage and forms the closing of the rib cage at the heart.

Observe Figure 180 and note how both the ribs and the clavicles connect to the sternum, completing the cagelike formation of the thorax. Figure 181 shows the formation from a side view, and Figure 182 shows the juncture of the ribs forming the sternum. The sternum is a pain-sensitive target. Using the thumb-knuckle fist illustrated in Chapter 1, strike your sternum with a low-medium force. Hard, pointed weapons, such as the two-

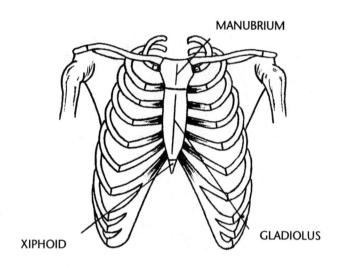

FIGURE 180

knuckle-focused straight-line punch, the knuckle-
focused backhand, and similar weapons, are also effective. Because of their potential power, all of the kicks
work well on this target as well.

THORACIC
VERTEBRAE

STERNUM

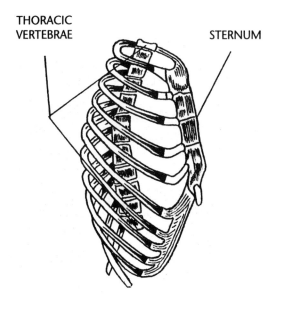

FIGURE 181

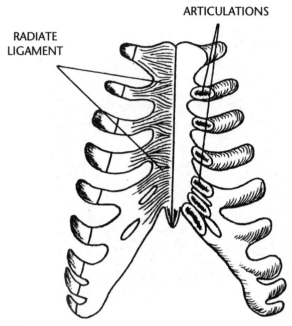

ARTICULATIONS

RADIATE
LIGAMENT

FIGURE 182

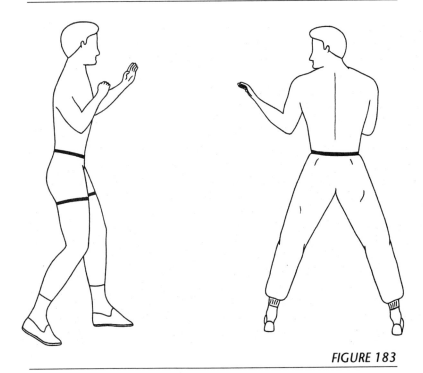

FIGURE 183

Practical Application Technique #36

In this first technique, you will be facing your opponent in a left forward straddle stance (fig. 183) to use a kicking defense. The spinning side kick that you will study here is one of the most powerful kicks in the martial arts.

As your opponent begins his advance, shift your weight forward onto your lead leg and chamber your right leg for a side kick (fig. 184). Rotate to your right and focus on your opponent with your peripheral vision, as in Figure 185, which shows the kick already en route to the target. Continue spinning your entire body and deliver your spinning side kick to your opponent's sternum (fig. 186). To accentuate the amount of penetration achieved with this kick, it is not locked out in the illustration. The completed kick requires the kicking leg to be fully locked into the open position. As you can

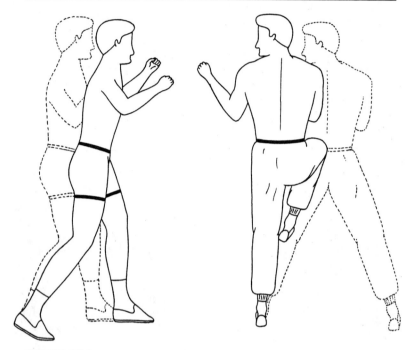

FIGURE 184

see from the position of the leg in the illustration, the
extended kick, if properly delivered, would send the
opponent sailing backward. A further analysis of this
kick can be found in *Da Qiang Ji: Power Striking*.

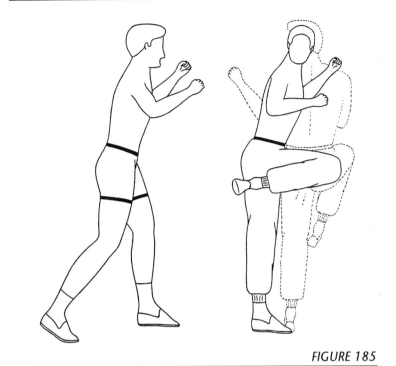

FIGURE 185

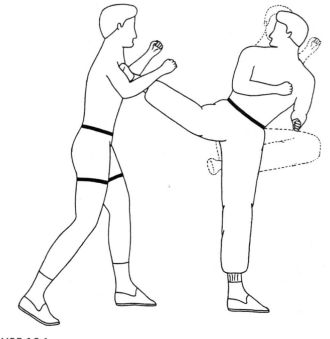

FIGURE 186

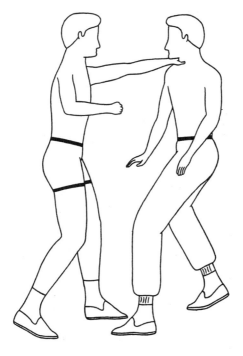

FIGURE 187

Practical Application Technique #37

This is a one-hand choke attack (fig. 187), and you will use a wrapping arm trap and a short straight-line punch combination. Look at where your hand is in Figure 187, then study Figure 188. To get to this point, rotate your right arm across your body to the left and make a wide clockwise circle with your arm reaching over your opponent's arm. Continue this rotation through the point where the back of your upper arm hits the choking arm just above the wrist. As you continue the rotation, your opponent's hand will be forced off your neck. At the completion of the clockwise circle, your right arm will be back to its starting position as illustrated in Figure 187, but your opponent's hand will be trapped under your arm. Keeping the arm down and pressed against your opponent's hand, raise your right hand and get a firm grip on his arm just above the

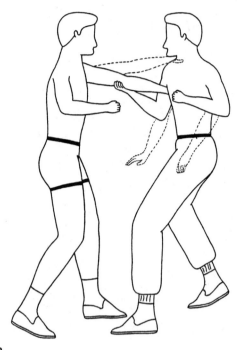

FIGURE 188

elbow. Chamber your left hand for a straight-line punch. Figure 189 illustrates a full-turn punch to the sternum. Note the difference in the shoulder positions of this illustration and Figure 188. As you lock this punch out, rotate your upper body into the stroke to maximize impact power.

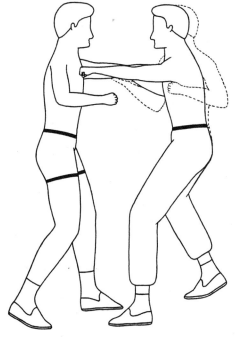

FIGURE 189

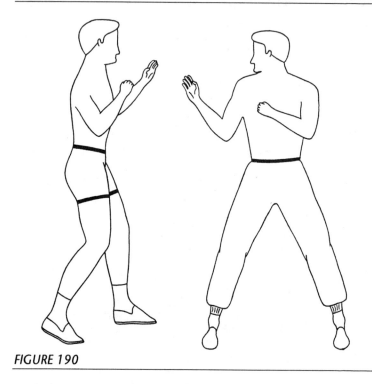

FIGURE 190

Practical Application Technique #38

In this technique you will be starting from a right-faced straddle stance, as in Figure 190. You will be moving to the inside of your opponent's right punch, so you will want to maintain visual contact with his left hand. As your opponent advances with his right punch (fig. 191), take a slight step to the rear of your stance, placing your right foot outside his left foot. Bring your right hand slightly toward your body as you contact the incoming punch with a crossing palm block. In Figure 192, your block is a flowing strike to your opponent's arm following an arc to the position shown. Shift your weight toward your right leg as you begin your counterstrike (fig. 193). Strike your opponent's sternum with a long-form backhand.

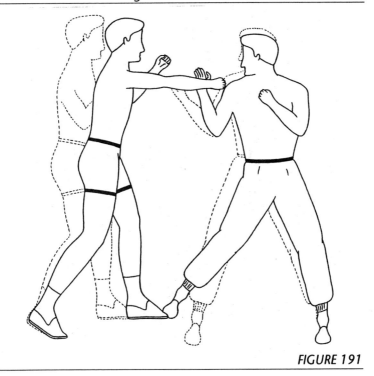

FIGURE 191

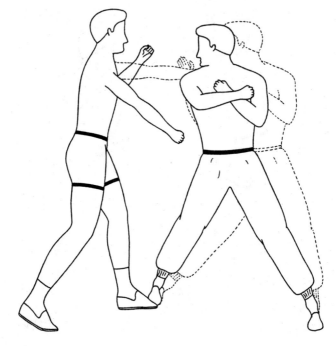

FIGURE 192

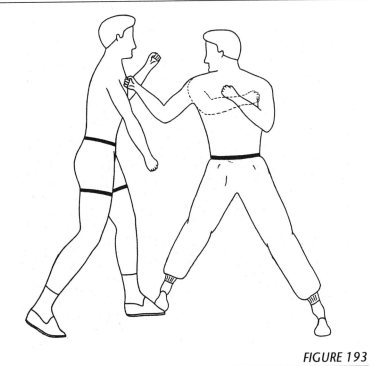

FIGURE 193

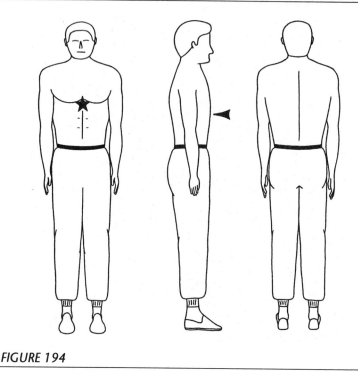

FIGURE 194

PRESSURE POINT #15: SOLAR PLEXUS

Figure 194 illustrates the location of your target area where the end of the sternum meets the abdominal muscles. To properly understand this pressure point and the effects of striking it, two basic contact centers must be analyzed.

To begin, the solar plexus is described as the epigastric and celiac plexus. The term solar plexus refers to the nerve network supplying all the viscera in the abdominal cavity. In this network exists a multitude of nerves and ganglia, as well as nine other plexuses. The nerve mass surrounds the celiac trunk and mesenetric artery above the abdominal aorta (fig. 195). Observe Figure 196. The principal ganglia of the solar plexus are the two semilunar ganglia located on either side of the plexus. They are the largest ganglia in the body and represent the basis for an attack to this pressure point.

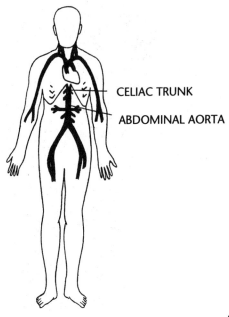

CELIAC TRUNK

ABDOMINAL AORTA

FIGURE 195

When the solar plexus is struck properly, the diaphragm contracts and is then paralyzed momentarily. The commonly used term for this reaction is "knocking the wind out" of someone, and it often causes unconsciousness for a brief period of time.

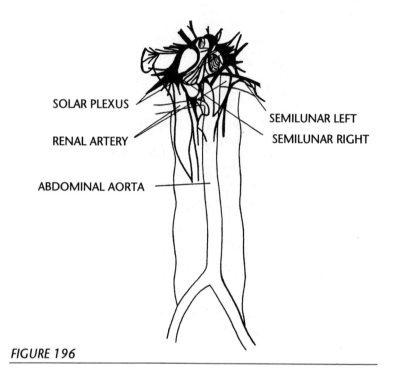

SOLAR PLEXUS

RENAL ARTERY

SEMILUNAR LEFT

SEMILUNAR RIGHT

ABDOMINAL AORTA

FIGURE 196

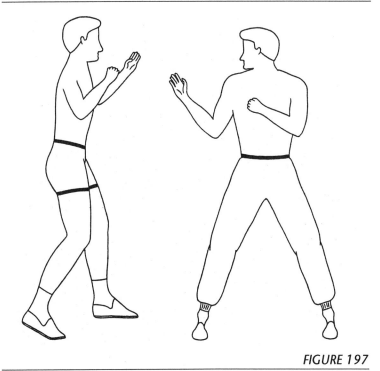

FIGURE 197

Practical Application Technique #39

You are positioned in a right-faced straddle stance, and your opponent is in a ready stance (fig. 197). In Figure 198, your opponent has advanced with a left vertical jab, and you have stepped outside the advancing punch and bumped it away with a right palm block. Your left arm is in the chamber position for a straight-arm centrifugal force strike. Using a thumb-knuckle fist, rotate your body clockwise, shuffle-step forward, and drive your counterstrike into your opponent's solar plexus, as in Figure 199.

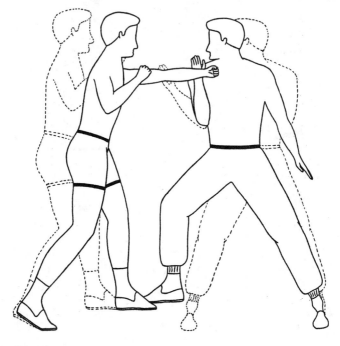

FIGURE 198

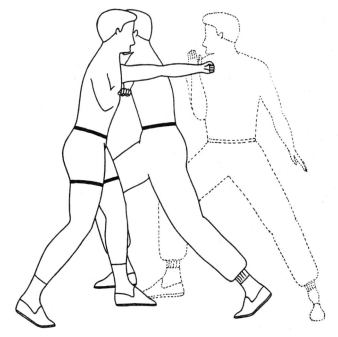

FIGURE 199

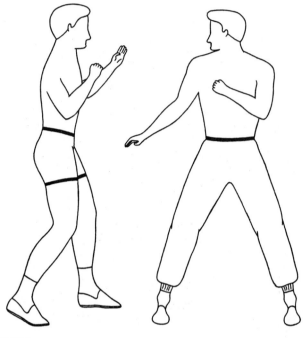

FIGURE 200

Practical Application Technique #40

Again you are positioned in a right forward straddle stance with your opponent in a standard ready position (fig. 200). Note the close proximity between you and your opponent. When you allow an opponent to get this close, you must be prepared for quick movement.

As your opponent advances with his punch (fig. 201), shift your body weight to your rear leg and chamber a right side kick. Figure 202 depicts your lock position; your target is, of course, the solar plexus. Portions of the opponent's anatomy have been omitted to show the depth of the penetration achieved with the kick from this distance. Note that the heel of the standing foot has rotated in the direction of the blow.

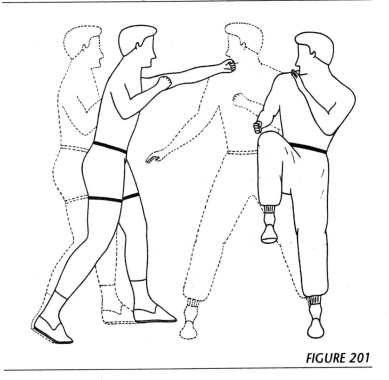

FIGURE 201

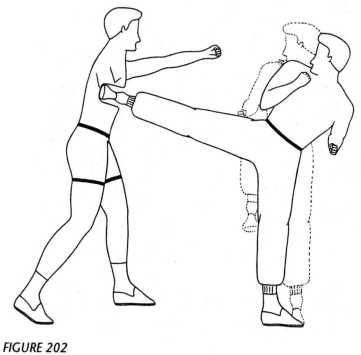

FIGURE 202

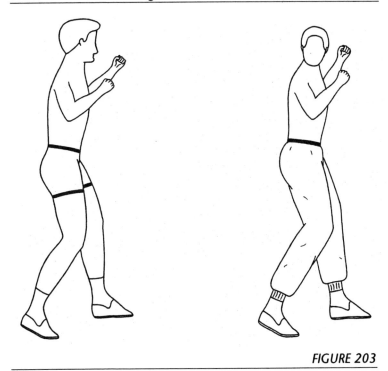

FIGURE 203

Practical Application Technique #41

In Figure 203, your opponent is advancing from your rear, and you will be defending yourself with a stationary back kick. As your opponent begins his advance, bring your weight forward onto your left foot and chamber your right leg for a back kick (fig. 204). In Figure 205, you drive your back kick into your opponent's solar plexus.

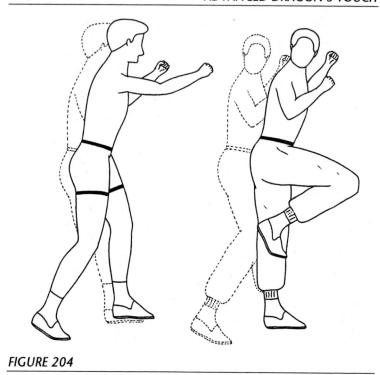

FIGURE 204

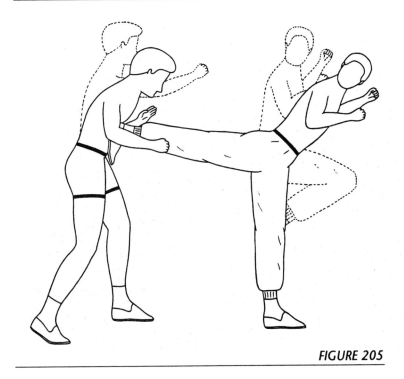

FIGURE 205

CHAPTER FIVE

Pressure Points #16 through #20

In this chapter, we will study the last set of five pressure points, which are as follows: the ribs, thoracic vertebrae, coccyx, median nerve, and elbow. As targets, the elbow and the median nerve are the types of pressure points that require skilled delivery of countermovements. A properly executed attack to the thoracic vertebrae and the coccyx can have long-term debilitating effects because of the proximity of these two targets to the spinal cord. An attack to the ribs, depending upon which ribs you attack and how your blow is delivered, can be a knockdown, a knockout, and possibly lethal.

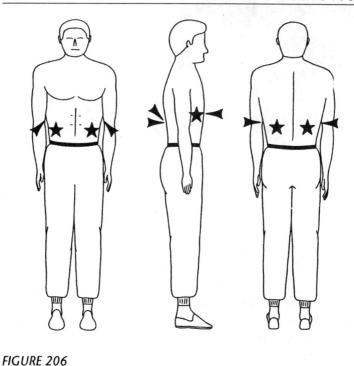

FIGURE 206

PRESSURE POINT #16: RIBS

Observe Figure 206. At first glance you will notice that all three figures have stars and arrows on them denoting points of attack. As discussed in the analyses of previous pressure points, the ribs form a protective cage for the heart and lungs, as well as forming the shape of the chest. The figure on the left denotes the lower sides of the ribs as targets as well as the "point" of the rib cage in the front. The point is so termed because the ribs seem to come to a point here, rising sharply and forming a tilted right angle after descending from the sternum. The center figure denotes those same areas as well as the twelfth ribs, and the figure on the right denotes the twelfth ribs and the ribs at the sides as targets.

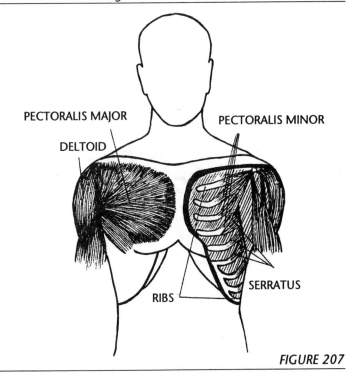

PECTORALIS MAJOR

PECTORALIS MINOR

DELTOID

SERRATUS

RIBS

FIGURE 207

Observe Figures 207 and 208. The twelfth ribs are sometimes referred to as the "short" or "floating" ribs. Note that they are unattached at their distal ends; this is what makes striking them so dangerous. You will note that the kidneys are directly behind these open-end ribs. If your blow contacts these ribs at the proper angle and is powerful enough to dislodge them from their position on the thoracic vertebrae or break them along their length, it is likely that the broken or dislodged bone would be forced into a kidney. The results would be similar to using a puncturing weapon on the kidney: immense pain quickly followed by death.

The "winding" effect is the most probable result of striking the ribs at the other indicated areas, but a compound-power or centrifugal-force blow applied to these areas could break them, sending shattered bones into the lungs. Because of the size of this target and its acces-

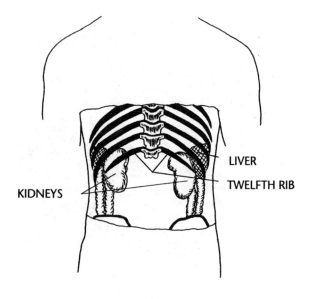

FIGURE 208

sibility to low kicks, it is considered a key target in technical fighting.

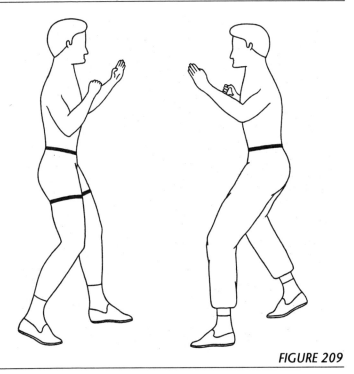

FIGURE 209

Practical Application Technique #42

Starting from a ready stance (fig. 209), you will be using a stationary block-and-strike technique designed to utilize a minimum of movement. As your opponent's straight right hand approaches (fig. 210), shift your weight to your rear leg and chamber your lead leg for a roundhouse kick. As you move back, apply a grappling palm block on the wrist of the incoming punch. Maintain your grip on the wrist of the punching arm and release a short roundhouse kick to your opponent's ribs, as in Figure 211.

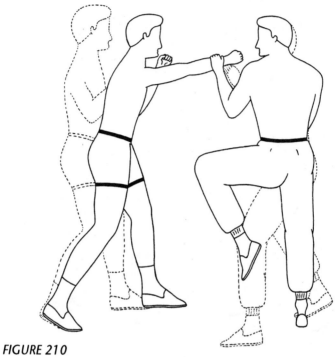

FIGURE 210

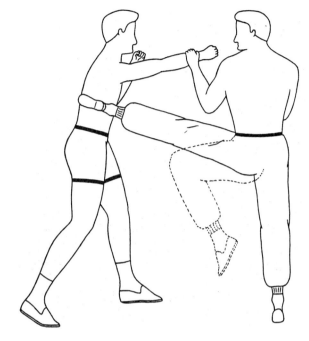

FIGURE 211

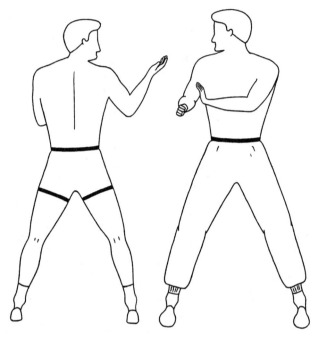

FIGURE 212

Practical Application Technique #43

We are going to use another grappling block and short kick, but beginning from a different stance (fig. 212). Position yourself in a right-faced straddle stance and be ready for a quick weight shift onto the rear leg. You have deliberately put yourself within hand range of your opponent. As your opponent snaps out a short right-side punch (fig. 213), shift your weight onto your back leg and chamber your right side kick. As you do this, catch the incoming punch with an outside suto block. Shifting the heel of the standing foot toward your opponent, snap out a short side kick to his ribs (fig. 214).

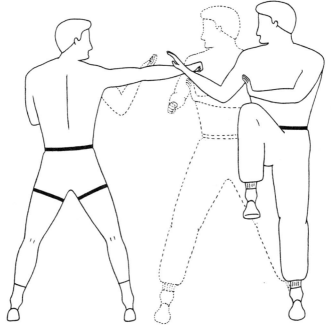

FIGURE 213

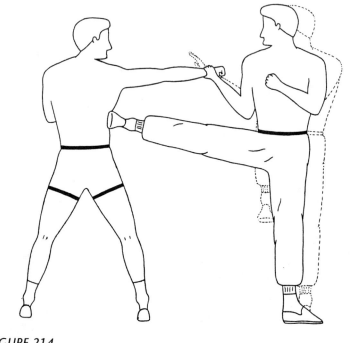

FIGURE 214

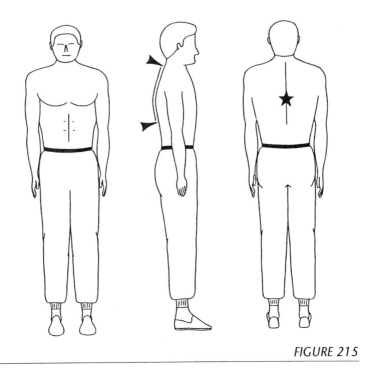

FIGURE 215

PRESSURE POINT #17: THORACIC SPINE

Observe Figure 215. The thoracic vertebrae are located along the line that appears in the third figure and are also indicated in the center figure. These vertebrae begin where the cervical vertebrae end and travel approximately three-quarters of the way down the back. As we have already discussed with pressure point #9 (cervical vertebrae), vertebrae provide support and attachment for other portions of the skeletal structure while creating a protected path for the descent of the spinal cord from the brain.

The cord passes through the hollowed area behind the vertebral bodies referred to in Figure 216. Five of the eight nerve roots that form the cardiac plexus protrude from the first five thoracic vertebrae, which means that attacks to this area have a direct effect on the heart,

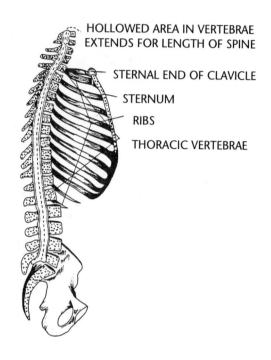

HOLLOWED AREA IN VERTEBRAE
EXTENDS FOR LENGTH OF SPINE

STERNAL END OF CLAVICLE

STERNUM

RIBS

THORACIC VERTEBRAE

FIGURE 216

which could range in severity from unconsciousness to
cardiac arrest. Powerful enough blows anywhere on this
structure will cause momentary paralysis below the
point of impact.

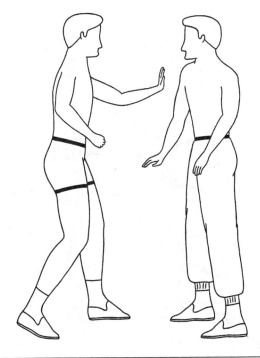

FIGURE 217

Practical Application Technique #44

In this technique, we will be defending against a common street attack, a push (fig. 217), and will be striking our designated target as a finishing maneuver.

As the pushing arm extends, take a deep step to the outside of the arm, clamp it with your right hand, and guide it past your body, as in Figure 218. Note the rotated position of your upper body. Pull the pushing arm down across your upper body and reach forward with your left hand (fig. 219), taking a grip on the back of your opponent's neck. As in Figure 220, release the pushing arm, push downward on your opponent's neck, and drive your left knee upward into your opponent's solar plexus. Raise your left arm in position for a downward elbow strike (fig. 221). Drive your elbow downward into your opponent's thoracic vertebrae while simultaneously dropping your weight

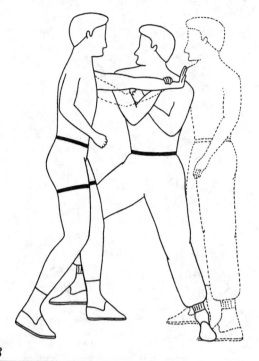

FIGURE 218

back down to enhance the power of your finishing blow (fig. 222).

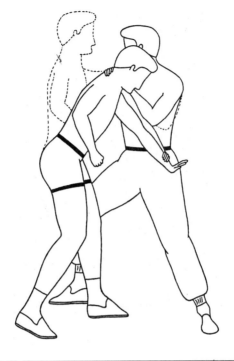

FIGURE 219

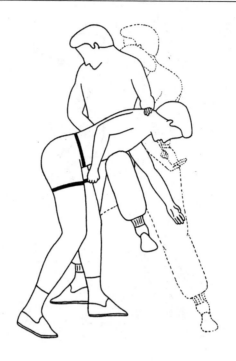

FIGURE 220

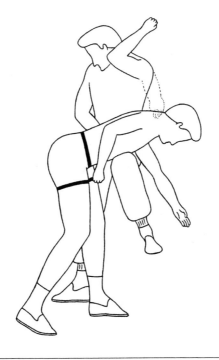

FIGURE 221

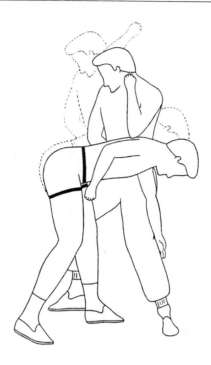

FIGURE 222

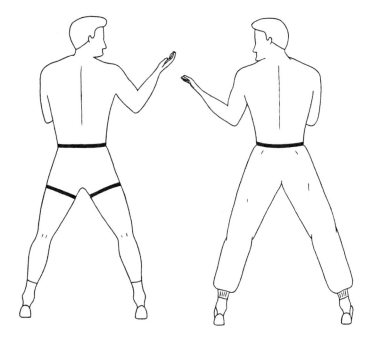

FIGURE 223

Practical Application Technique #45

When an opponent commits his body into a reaching stroke, he must then make whatever recovery movements are necessary to maintain his balance before being able to initiate another efficient stroke. During such attacks, you are able to initiate more time-consuming counterstrikes, such as will be used here.

Begin in the side straddle position shown (fig. 223). In Figure 224, your opponent has lunged toward you with a reaching backhand. To reach this position, push off and take a rearward step with the left foot, pivot the right foot as shown, and shift all of your weight onto the left foot. Rotate your upper body and turn your head over your right shoulder, bringing your opponent within the span of your peripheral vision. Now, as in Figures 225 and 226, raise your right foot and extend the corresponding leg while

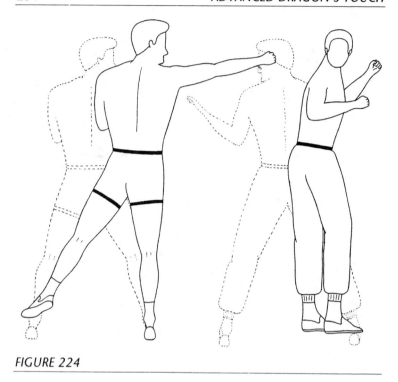

FIGURE 224

continuing the rotation of your body and strike the
thoracic vertebrae with your hook kick.

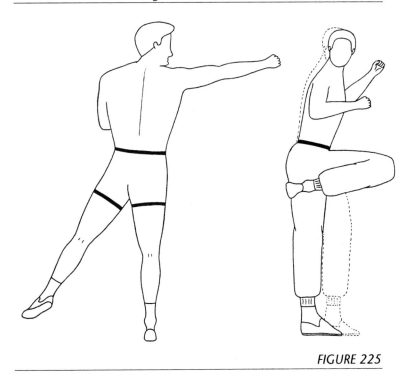

FIGURE 225

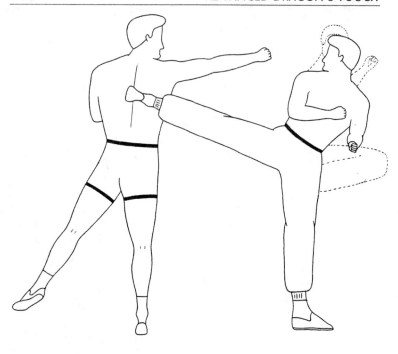

FIGURE 226

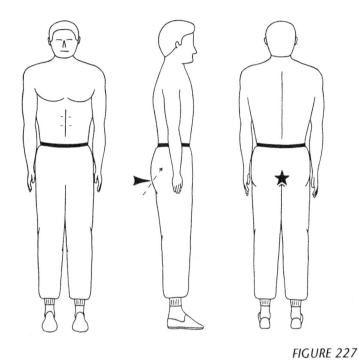

FIGURE 227

PRESSURE POINT #18: COCCYX

You could not possibly imagine the paralyzing pain of being hit in the coccyx without having experienced it. A neural shock is immediately felt through the length of the spine and into the back of the head, as well as through the limbs. The stroke must be precise, but, again, your attack here is spinal, which involves neurological responses and could cause partial permanent paralysis of the lower extremities.

In Figure 227, the center and right figures denote your point of attack, and the dotted arrow in the center figure depicts the angle of attack required to strike the coccyx effectively. Observe Figure 228. The coccyx, also called the tailbone, comprises three small vetebrae affixed to the tip of the sacrum. The blow to this area should make contact between the buttocks just above the anus.

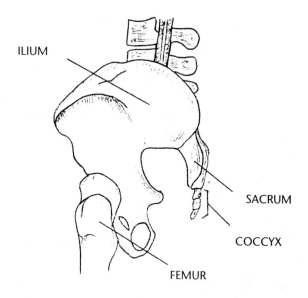

ILIUM

SACRUM

COCCYX

FEMUR

FIGURE 228

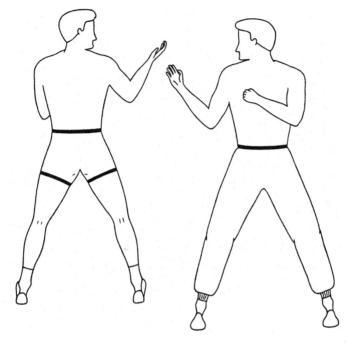

FIGURE 229

Practical Application Technique #46

Both you and your opponent start out in right-faced side-straddle positions (fig. 229). Be prepared for a quick backward movement. In Figure 230, your opponent has lunged at you with a long backhand. Shift your weight to the rear leg and raise your right foot slightly. Block the incoming backhand with a suto block just as you shift your balance to your left leg. The rising hook kick in Figure 231 should make contact with the coccyx at the angle depicted in the center in Figure 227.

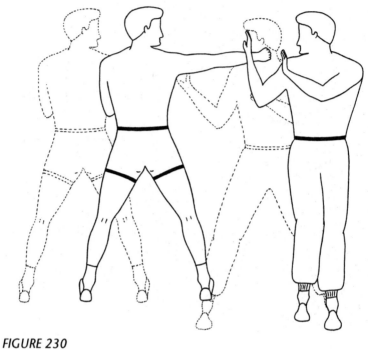

FIGURE 230

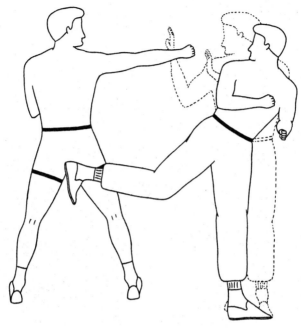

FIGURE 231

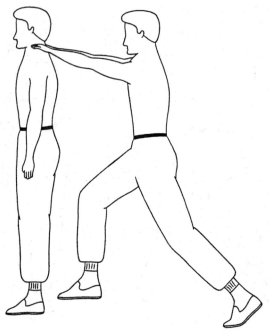

FIGURE 232

Practical Application Technique #47

Observe Figures 232 and 233. This rising knee stroke approaches the coccyx at a near-perfect angle. Take a grip on your opponent's shoulders and drive your knee forward and upward into his coccyx.

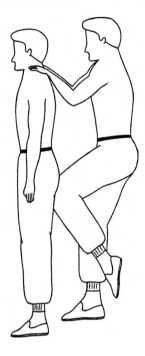

FIGURE 233

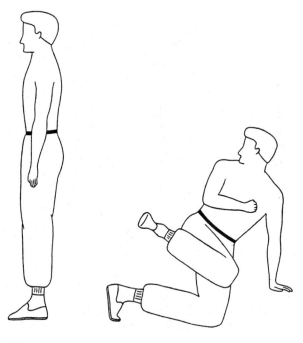

FIGURE 234

Practical Application Technique #48

The side kick shown in Figures 234 and 235 closely parallels the form of the aerial side kick and uses the standard lock/snap thrust characteristic of all side kicks. In delivering this kick, drive the heel of your foot into the target area.

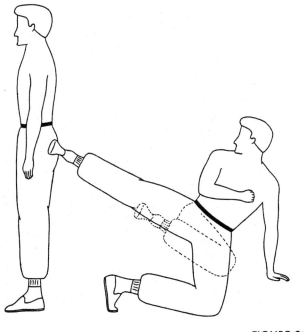

FIGURE 235

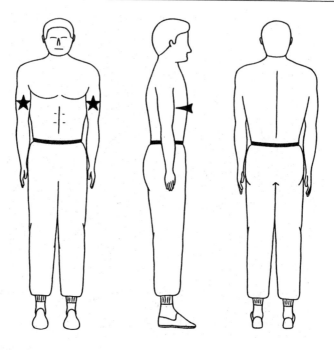

FIGURE 236

PRESSURE POINT #19: MEDIAN NERVE

The median nerve is exposed to attack almost every time the arm is used, and because of the debilitating effect of striking it, this is an ideal target when your intention is to end a confrontation without inflicting a great deal of damage.

The first and center illustrations in Figure 236 denote your target area. Figures 237 through 239 show a subsurface view of the target, progressively removing layers of muscle until the nerves are exposed in Figure 239. As this illustration depicts, the median nerve is a lower branch of the brachial plexus. Striking this pressure point is extremely painful and will temporarily paralyze the corresponding arm, rendering it completely useless for several minutes.

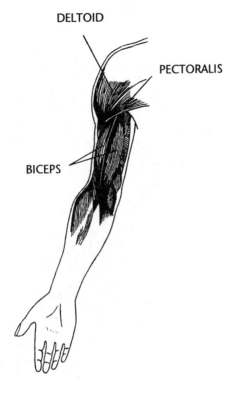

DELTOID

PECTORALIS

BICEPS

FIGURE 237

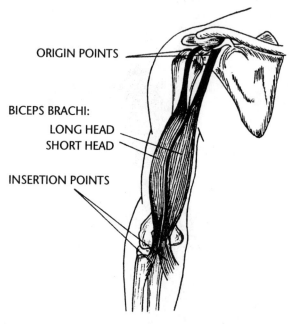

FIGURE 238

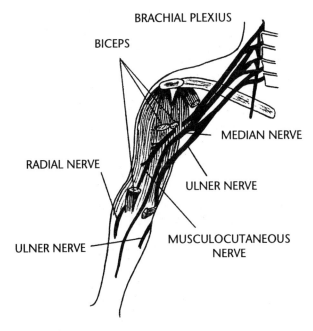

FIGURE 239

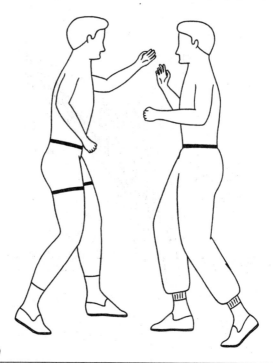

FIGURE 240

Practical Application Technique #49

Only one technique will be taught with this pressure
point, and it is intended as an example to inspire cre-
ativity. Suto, hammer, backhand, vertical and full-turn
punches, and even elbows can be used against this area.
As long as the weapon has a solid contact point and is
applied with maximum penetration, the blow will yield
the expected results.

Figure 240 is a modified ready stance. Note that
your right leg is in the lead position and that both
hands are held low on the torso. Your opponent is
reaching out to slap or grab. As in Figure 241, step
back into a forward stance and apply an inside suto
block to the approaching hand. As you do this, chamber a left suto. With your blocking hand, take a grip
on your opponent's wrist and rotate his arm into a
palm-up position (fig. 242). Finally, deliver a full

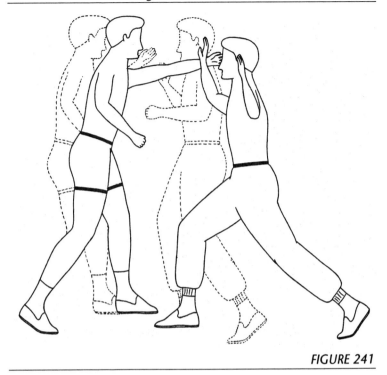

FIGURE 241

downward vertical suto to your opponent's median
nerve (fig. 243).

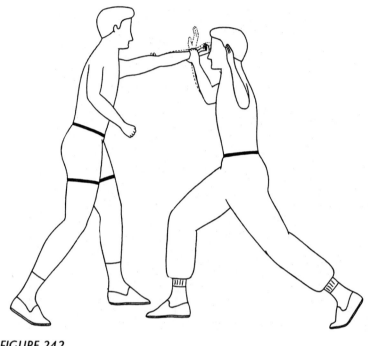

FIGURE 242

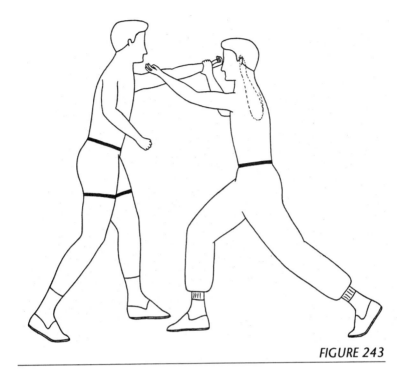

FIGURE 243

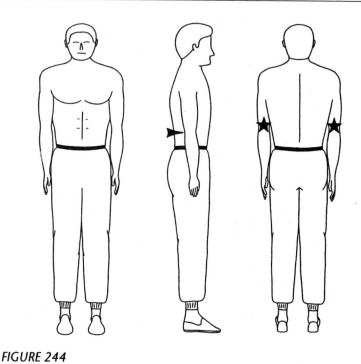

FIGURE 244

PRESSURE POINT #20: THE ELBOW

Targeting the elbow as a pressure point requires skilled technical movement. In this text we have used this same area as a weapon, so it is obvious that the elbow is not simply a fragile area. However, applying pressure to the elbow when the arm is extended changes its strength considerably. The target area is pointed out in Figure 244.

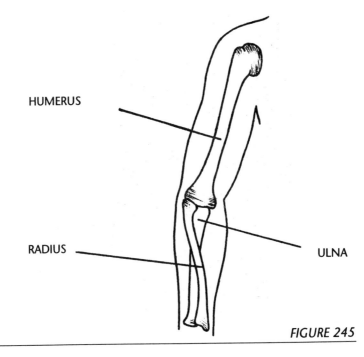

HUMERUS

RADIUS

ULNA

FIGURE 245

Observe Figures 245 and 246. The elbow is the junction of the humerus, radius, and ulna. The bone of the upper arm is a single structure. Two bones, the radius and the ulna, occupy the lower arm, and, as the illustrations depict, they cross or run parallel according to the position of the hand. When the hand is faced palm up, the radius and the ulna run parallel; when the hand is faced palm down, the radius crosses over the ulna.

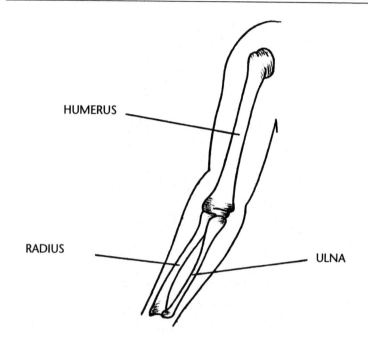

FIGURE 246

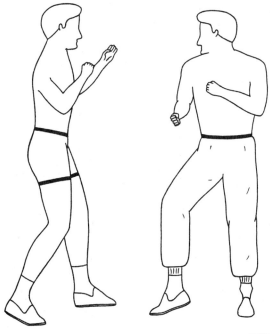

FIGURE 247

Practical Application Technique #50

Figure 247 depicts a cat stance with the hands held low on the torso to draw a punch to the face. As your opponent advances with his straight right punch (fig. 248), you step to the inside of the blow and execute a double hammer block. Your left hand makes contact with medium pressure, while your right hand executes a horizontal strike to the median nerve by using the blocking area of your arm as a weapon. Immediately turn your right hand over as in Figure 249, open it to a palm strike, and deliver a rising palm strike to your opponent's nose while taking a full grip on his wrist with your left hand and rotating his arm palm up. In Figure 250, you drop your right arm down and lock it in the extended position. Now, in a simultaneous motion, pull down the wrist and drive your right arm upward, striking your opponent's elbow (fig. 251).

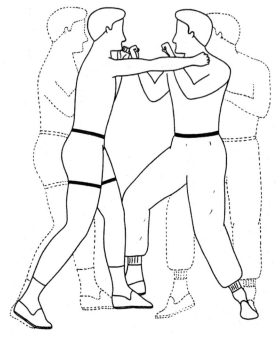

FIGURE 248

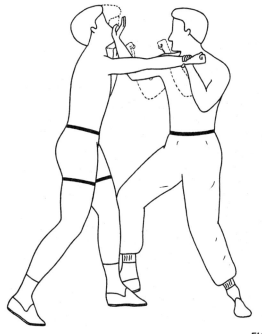

FIGURE 249

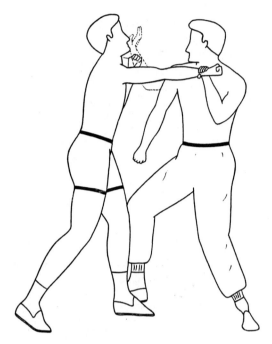

FIGURE 250

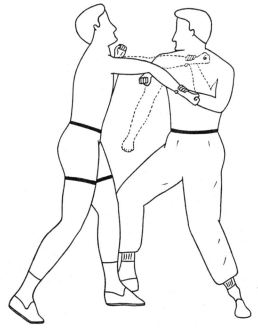

FIGURE 251

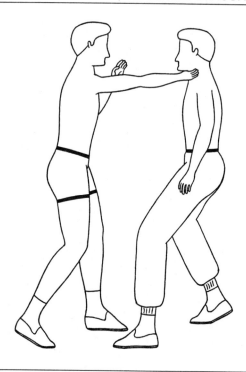

FIGURE 252

Practical Application Technique #51

In Figure 252, your opponent has grabbed you in a one-hand choke with his arm locked, an ideal position for elbow-breaking techniques. With both hands working simultaneously, drive your palms into the inside of his arm above the wrist and into the outside of his arm at the elbow, as in Figures 253 and 254.

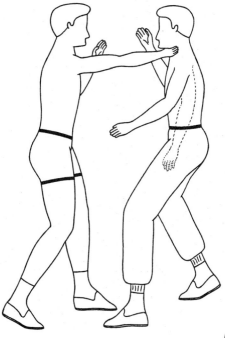

FIGURE 253

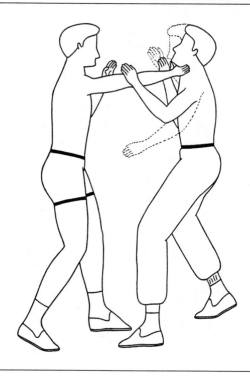

FIGURE 254

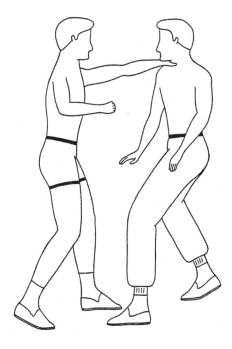

FIGURE 255

Practical Application Technique #52

We are again starting from a one-hand choke, this time with the left hand (fig. 255). Look closely at the arm positions in Figures 256 and 257. From your starting position in Figure 255, rotate the extended arm clockwise across your body and pull your head back just as your upper arm makes contact with your opponent's wrist. Note that your left hand is rising into a palm-up position. Note also that your opponent's wrist is trapped under your armpit. Take a strong grip on your opponent's elbow with your left hand and lay your right hand directly over your left (fig. 258). While leaning back with your upper body, drive your palms upward, snapping the elbow (fig. 259). Be careful when practicing with a training partner; this technique is very effective.

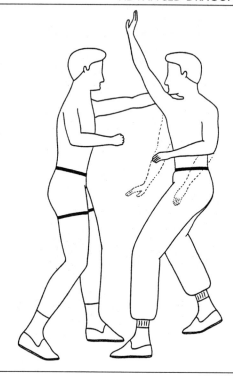

FIGURE 256

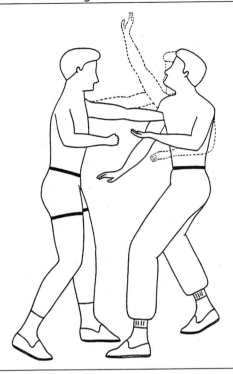

FIGURE 257

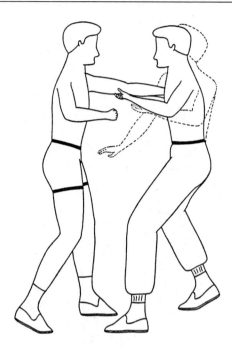

FIGURE 258

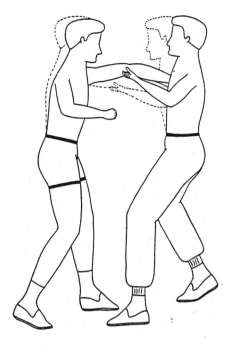

FIGURE 259